Atlas of Musculoskeletal Ultrasound Anatomy

Second Edition

Atlas of Musculoskeletal Ultrasound Anatomy

Second Edition

Dr Mike Bradley, FRCR
Consultant Radiologist,
North Bristol NHS Trust,
Honorary Senior Lecturer,
University of Bristol

Dr Paul O'Donnell, FRCR
Consultant Radiologist,
Royal National Orthopaedic Hospital,
Stanmore, Middlesex,
Honorary Senior Lecturer,
University College,
London

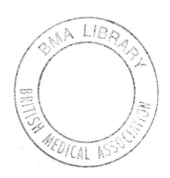

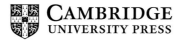

CAMBRIDGE UNIVERSITY PRESS
Cambridge, New York, Melbourne, Madrid, Cape Town, Singapore,
São Paulo, Delhi, Dubai, Tokyo

Cambridge University Press
The Edinburgh Building, Cambridge CB2 8RU, UK

Published in the United States of America by
Cambridge University Press, New York

www.cambridge.org
Information on this title: www.cambridge.org/9780521728096

First published 2010

Printed in the United Kingdom at the University Press, Cambridge

*A catalogue record for this publication is available from the
British Library*

Library of Congress Cataloguing-in-Publication Data

Bradley, Mike, Dr.
  Atlas of musculoskeletal ultrasound anatomy / Mike Bradley,
Paul O'Donnell. – 2nd ed.
    p. ; cm.
  Includes index.
  ISBN 978-0-521-72809-6 (pbk.)
    1. Musculoskeletal system–Ultrasonic imaging. 2. Musculoskeletal
system–Diseases–Diagnosis–Atlases. 3. Ultrasonic imaging–Atlases.
I. O'Donnell, Paul. II. Title.
    [DNLM: 1. Musculoskeletal System–anatomy & histology–
Atlases. 2. Musculoskeletal System–ultrasonography–Atlases.
3. Musculoskeletal Diseases–ultrasonography–Atlases.
WE 17 B8105d 2010]
  RC925.7.B73 2010
  616.7'07548–dc22
                                                    2009034805

ISBN 978-0-521-72809-6 Paperback

Contents

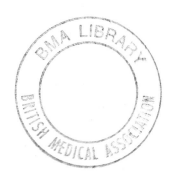

Foreword

The quality of ultrasonic images has seen radical improvement over the last couple of years, and – as can be appreciated in the new edition of this *Atlas of Musculoskeletal Ultrasound Anatomy* – high frequency applications such as musculoskeletal ultrasound have profited from this development.

Significant advances in ultrasonic probe design and refined manufacturing techniques have resulted in transducers with outstandingly high bandwidth and sensitivity to provide ultrasonic images with both excellent spatial resolution and penetration at the same time. State-of-the-art transducer technology also boosts Doppler performance and supports advanced imaging functions such as trapezoid scan for an extended field of view at no loss of spatial resolution. High frequency matrix transducers make use of genuine 4-D imaging technology to achieve finer and more uniform ultrasonic beams in all three dimensions to deliver the most superb and artefact-free images from the very near to the far field.

Also the dramatic increase of processing power in premium ultrasound systems such as the Aplio XG, with which most of the cases described in this book were acquired, has triggered a quantum leap in image quality. Advanced platforms can process the amount of data worth one DVD each second, which allows us to implement the most complex signal processing algorithms to improve image quality, suppress artefacts and extract the desired information from the ultrasonic raw data in real time.

Uncompromised image quality remains the fundamental merit and to support this in obtaining the fastest and best informed disease management decisions, a *variety* of powerful imaging functions such as Differential Tissue Harmonics, Advanced Dynamic Flow *or* Precision Imaging have been developed. *ApliPure+* real-time compounding, for example, can simultaneously perform spatial and frequency compounding in transmit and receive to enhance both image clarity and detail definition while preserving clinically significant markers such as shadows behind echo-dense objects. These advanced imaging functions work hand in hand with each other to provide the highest resolution and the finest detail. Naturally, they can be combined with virtually any other imaging mode such as colour Doppler or 3D/4D for even greater uniformity within each application.

In spite of all this technical development, we must not forget that the result of an ultrasound scan is highly dependent on the examiner's skills. Only the combination of technological excellence with the dedication and expertise of ultrasound enthusiasts such as the authors of this atlas makes ultrasonic images of outstanding diagnostic value as shown in this book a reality.

Joerg Schlegel

Principles and pitfalls of musculoskeletal ultrasound

High resolution – best results are obtained using a high frequency linear probe on a matched ultrasound system. Power Doppler is often helpful for pathological diagnosis as well as in the identification of normal anatomy.

Anisotropy – this phenomenon produces focal areas of hypo-echogenicity when the probe is not at 90° to the linear structure being imaged. This is particularly noticeable when imaging tendons resulting in simulation of hypo-echoic pathological lesions within the tendon. The sonographer can compensate for this by maintaining the 90° angle or by using compound imaging.

Anatomy – knowledge of the relevant anatomy is essential for accurate diagnosis and location of disease.

Symmetry – The sonographer can often compare anatomical areas for symmetry helping to diagnose subtle echographic changes.

Dynamic – ultrasound successfully lends itself to scanning whilst moving the relevant anatomy, either passive or resistive. This can help to demonstrate abnormalities which may be accentuated by movement.

Palpation – the sonographer has the opportunity to palpate the abnormality or anatomy linking the imaging directly with the symptomatology, in a manner not possible with other types of cross-sectional imaging.

Echogenicity of tissues

Echogenicity may vary somewhat with different ultrasound probe frequencies and machine set-up. This section describes these tissues using the common musculoskeletal presets and high frequency transducers. Surrounding tissue also influences echogenicity due to beam attenuation.

Fat – pure fat is hypo-echoic/transonic but the echogenicity varies in different anatomy and pathology. Fatty tumours such as lipomas contain areas of connective tissue creating the characteristic linear hyper-echoic lines parallel to the skin. Other fatty areas may vary in echogenicity depending on their structure and surrounding tissue.

Muscle – muscle fibres are hypo-echoic separated by hyper-echoic interfaces. Hyper-echoic fascia surrounds each muscle belly delineating the muscle groups.

Fascia – hyper-echoic thin, well-marginated soft tissue boundaries.

Tendon – the hyper-echoic tendon consists of interdigitated parallel fibres running in the long axis of the tendon. The tendon sheath is hyper-echoic separated from the tendon by a thin hypo-echoic area.

Para-tenon – some tendons do not have a true tendon sheath but are surrounded by an hyper-echoic boundary, the para-tenon, e.g. the Tendo-achilles.

Ligament – hyper-echoic, similar to tendons. Fibrillar pattern may vary in multilayered ligaments.

Synovium/Capsule – these structures around joints are not usually separately distinguishable on ultrasound, both appearing hypo-echoic and similar to joint fluid.

Hyaline cartilage – hypo-echoic/transonic cartilage is seen against highly reflective cortical bone.

Costal cartilage – hypo-echoic well defined. Well marginated from the hyper-echoic anterior rib end. The echogenicity varies depending on how much calcification it contains.

Fibrocartilage – hyper-echoic triangular-shaped cartilage with often internal specular echoes, e.g. the menisci.

Bone/Periosteum – this is indistinguishable in normal bone. Highly reflective hyper-echoic linear/curvi-linear line with acoustic shadowing.

Pleura – hyper-echoic parietal pleura is usually seen in the normal intercostal area. Aerated lung deep to this.

Air/gas – this is also highly reflective and creates characteristic 'comet tail' artefacts. Small gas bubbles in tissue may give small hyper-echoic foci whilst aerated lung is diffusely hyper-echoic with comet tails.

Nerve – hypo-echoic linear nerve bundles separated by hyper-echoic interfaces: appearances similar to tendons.

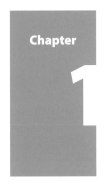

Chapter

1

Chest and neck

Supraclavicular fossa

This is an ill-defined area at the inferior aspect of the posterior triangle of the neck. It is bounded by the clavicle inferiorly, sternomastoid muscle medially and trapezius postero-laterally. The floor is muscular, comprising levator scapulae, splenius and the three scalene muscles.

Contents

- Accessory nerve
- Omohyoid
- External jugular vein
- Lymph nodes
- Subclavian artery
- Brachial plexus

Scalene muscles

Scalenus anterior
- Origin: anterior tubercles cervical vertebrae 3–6.
- Insertion: scalene tubercle first rib.

Scalenus medius
- Origin: posterior tubercles cervical vertebrae 2–7.
- Insertion: first rib, posterior to subclavian groove.

Scalenus posterior
- Origin: as part of scalenus medius.
- Insertion: second rib.

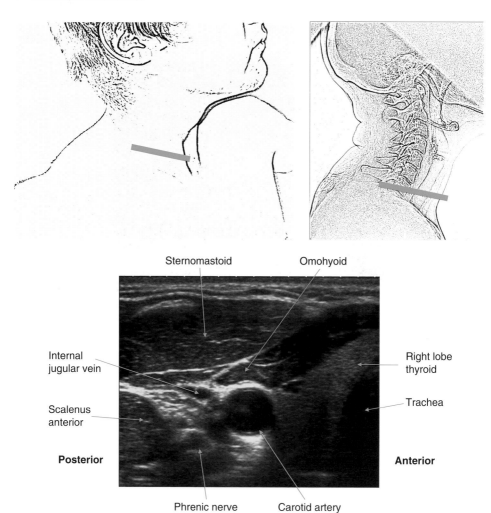

Fig. 1.1. Surface and radiographic anatomy of the sternomastoid. TS, anterior supraclavicular fossa, probe over sternomastoid.

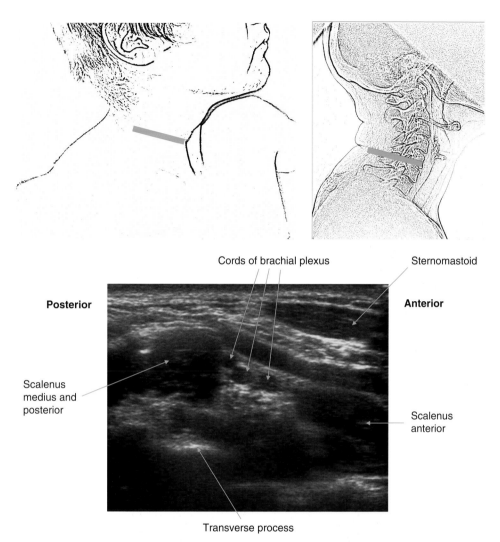

Posterior

Cords of brachial plexus

Sternomastoid

Anterior

Scalenus
medius and
posterior

Scalenus
anterior

Transverse process

Fig. 1.2. Surface and radiographic anatomy of the proximal brachial plexus. TS, supraclavicular fossa, probe on posterior sternomastoid.

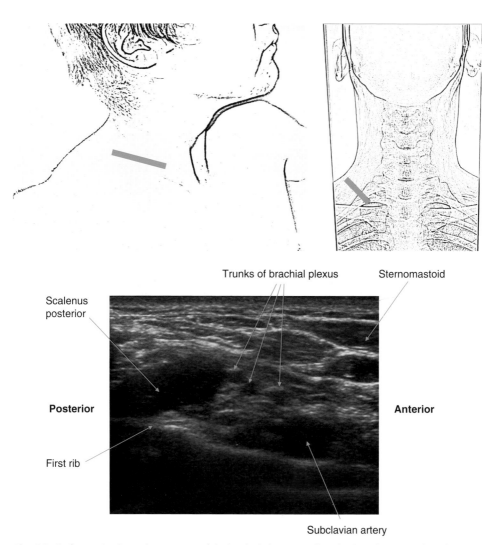

Fig. 1.3. Surface and radiographic anatomy of the brachial plexus over first rib. TS, probe postero-lateral to sternomastoid.

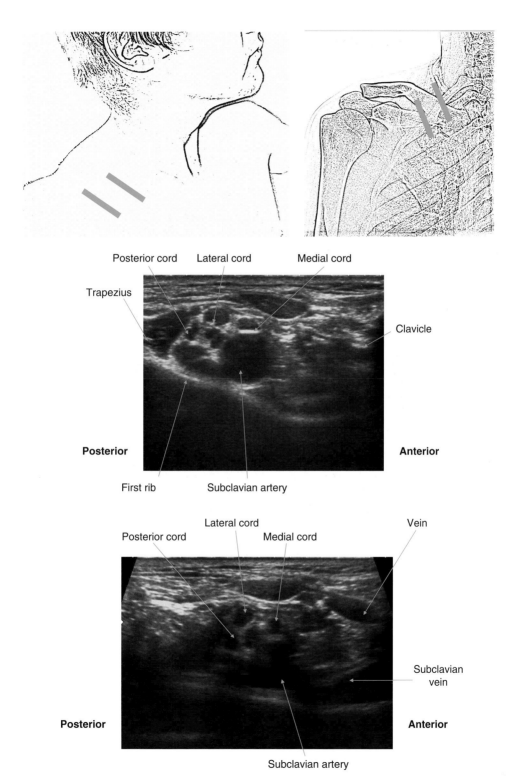

Fig. 1.4. Surface and radiographic anatomy of the distal brachial plexus. TS, probe superior to the mid/distal clavicle.

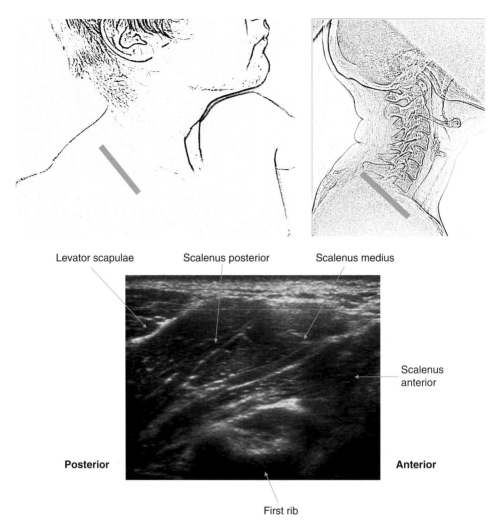

Fig. 1.5. Surface and radiographic anatomy of the scalene muscles. TS, posterior supraclavicular fossa.

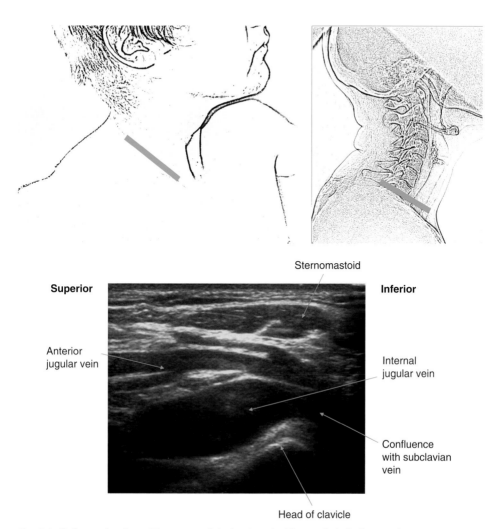

Fig. 1.6. Surface and radiographic anatomy of the jugular vein. LS, supraclavicular fossa, probe over posterior sternomastoid.

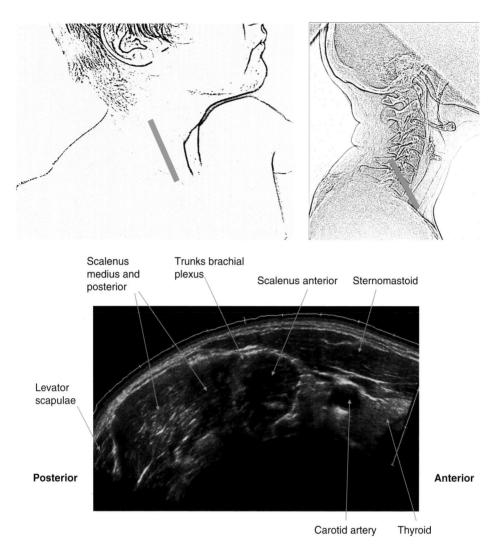

Fig. 1.7. Surface and radiographic anatomy of the supraclavicular fossa. Panorama supraclavicular fossa.

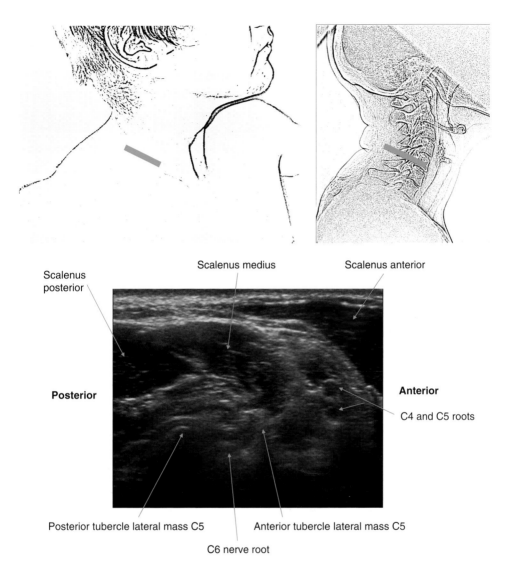

Fig. 1.8. Surface and radiographic anatomy of the C6 nerve root foramen (largest anterior and posterior tubercles of the lateral mass.) TS, probe over base lateral neck.

Infraclavicular fossa

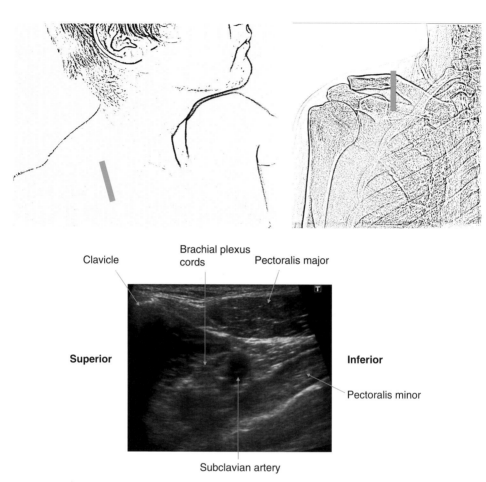

Clavicle

Brachial plexus cords

Pectoralis major

Superior

Inferior

Pectoralis minor

Subclavian artery

Fig. 1.9. Surface and radiographic anatomy of the infraclavicular fossa.

TS infraclavicular fossa

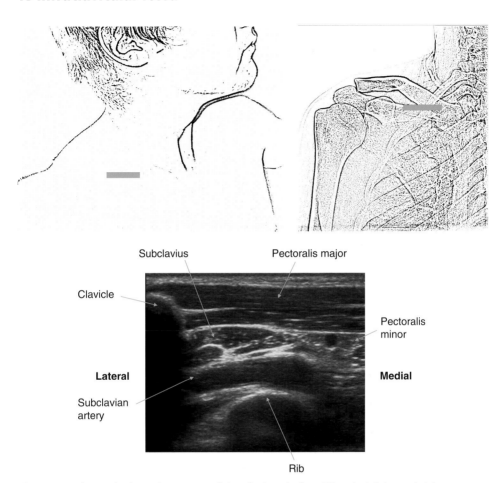

Fig. 1.10. Surface and radiographic anatomy of the infraclavicular fossa. TS, probe inferior to clavicle.

Sternoclavicular joint

This is an atypical synovial joint, like the acromioclavicular joint, as the articular surfaces are covered with fibrocartilage. The medial end of the clavicle articulates with the manubrium and first costal cartilage. The capsule is thickened anteriorly and posteriorly to form the sternoclavicular ligaments. Further ligaments attach to the first rib and contralateral clavicle.

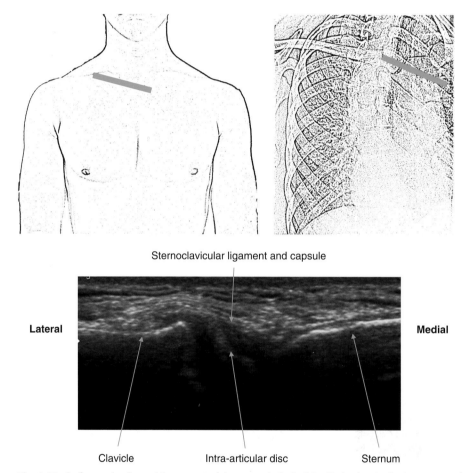

Fig. 1.11. Surface and radiographic anatomy of the sternoclavicular joint. Probe, longitudinal to joint, angled at 45 degrees.

Chest wall

Anterior

The thoracic wall muscles lie in three layers analogous to those in the abdomen, but separated by ribs. The outer two layers (external and internal intercostal) are usually visible in a rib space, deep to which can be seen the pleural space and lung. The neurovascular bundle lies deep to the second layer at the superior aspect of the intercostal space.

Ribs and costal cartilages

The anterior aspect of a rib articulates with a costal cartilage via a cartilaginous joint at which no movement is possible. The rib is deeply concave, and cartilage convex. The second to seventh costal cartilages articulate with the sternum via synovial joints. Calcification within costal cartilages is highly variable, and causes foci of hyperechogenicity.

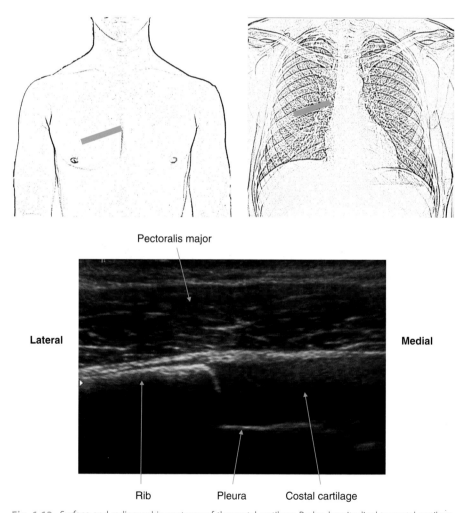

Fig. 1.12. Surface and radiographic anatomy of the costal cartilage. Probe, longitudinal to costal cartilage.

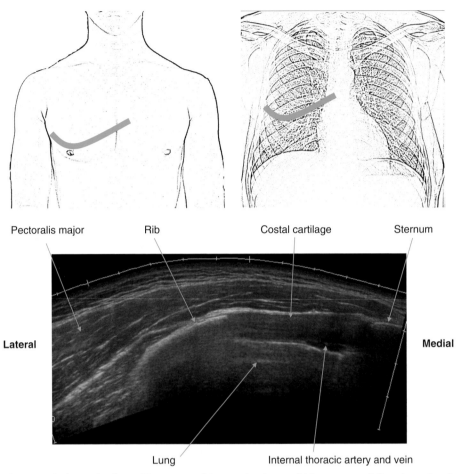

Fig. 1.13. Surface and radiographic anatomy of the anterior chest wall. LS, panorama of rib and costal cartilage.

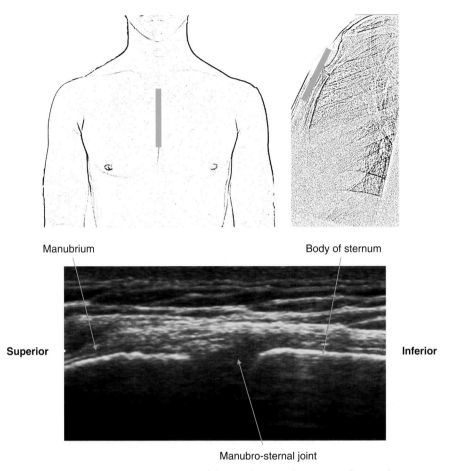

Manubrium

Body of sternum

Superior

Inferior

Manubro-sternal joint

Fig. 1.14. Surface and radiographic anatomy of the manubriosternal joint. LS, probe over the sternum.

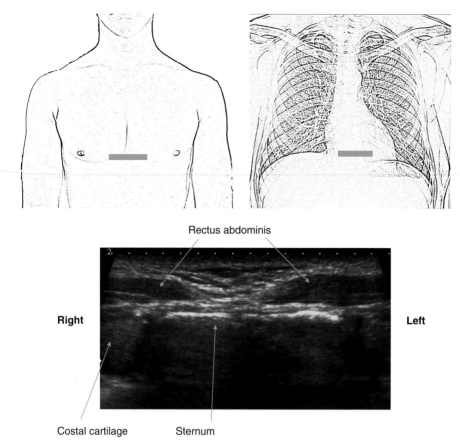

Fig. 1.15. Surface and radiographic anatomy of the Rectus abdominis insertion. TS, probe over lower anterior chest wall midline.

Lateral chest wall

External and internal intercostals
- Origin: lower border of superior rib.
- Insertion: upper border of inferior rib. Internal intercostals deep to external.

Serratus anterior
- Origin: upper eight ribs, overlying the lateral chest wall.
- Insertion: inferior angle and costal margin of the scapula. It forms the medial wall of the axilla.

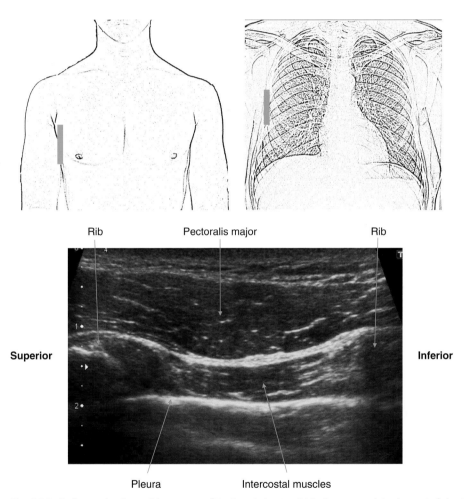

Fig. 1.16. Surface and radiographic anatomy of the lateral chest wall. LS, rib space on lateral aspect of chest.

Posterior chest wall

Trapezius muscle covers the posteromedial aspect of the upper chest.

- Origin: from skull to the T12 vertebra in the midline.
- Insertion: clavicle, acromion and spine of the scapula.

Deep to trapezius are the muscles that extend from the vertebral column to the medial aspect of the scapula – levator scapulae superiorly and the rhomboids inferiorly. Inferiorly, trapezius covers the superior aspect of latissimus dorsi. The erector spinae muscles are deep to the rhomboids.

Levator scapulae

- Origin: posterior tubercles of transverse processes of upper four cervical vertebrae.
- Insertion: superior angle, medial border of scapula.

Rhomboids

- Origin: lower part of ligamentum nuchae and spines of cervical and upper five thoracic vertebrae.
- Insertion: medial border scapula, major inferiorly, and minor between levator scapulae and major.

Latissimus dorsi

- Origin: spines of lower six thoracic vertebrae, lumbar fascia, lower four ribs and posterior iliac crest.
- Insertion: inferior angle of scapula.

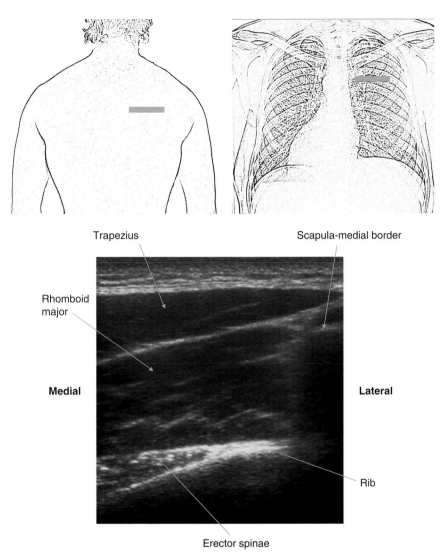

Trapezius

Scapula-medial border

Rhomboid
major

Medial

Lateral

Rib

Erector spinae

Fig. 1.17. Surface and radiographic anatomy of the posterior chest wall. TS, posterior chest wall, probe at medial border of scapula.

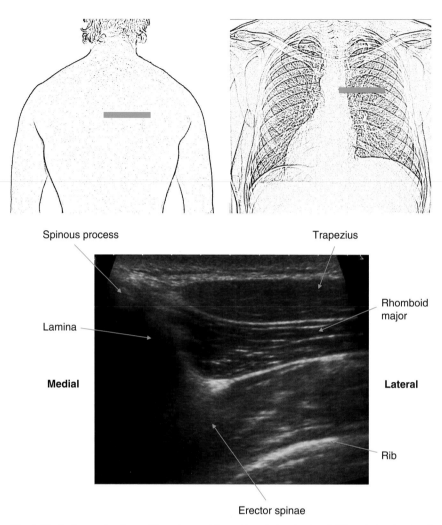

Fig. 1.18. Surface and radiographic anatomy of the mid posterior chest wall. TS, posterior chest wall, probe on spinous process.

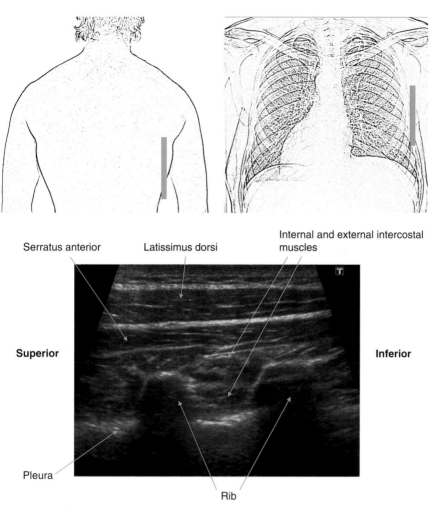

Fig. 1.19. Surface and radiographic anatomy of the intercostal muscles. LS, postero-lateral chest wall.

Axilla

This pyramidal space contains important neurovascular structures (axillary vessels and the cords of the brachial plexus), and lymph nodes. It communicates at its apex with the posterior triangle of the neck.

- Anterior wall: anterior axillary fold containing pectoralis major, pectoralis minor, subclavius.
- Posterior wall: subscapularis, latissimus dorsi and teres major from above downwards.
- Medial wall: serratus anterior and underlying chest wall.
- Lateral wall: bicipital groove of humerus.

The clavicle, scapula and the outer aspect of the first rib form the apex.

Subscapularis

- Origin: medial two-thirds of the costal surface of the scapula.
- Insertion: lesser tuberosity of the humerus.

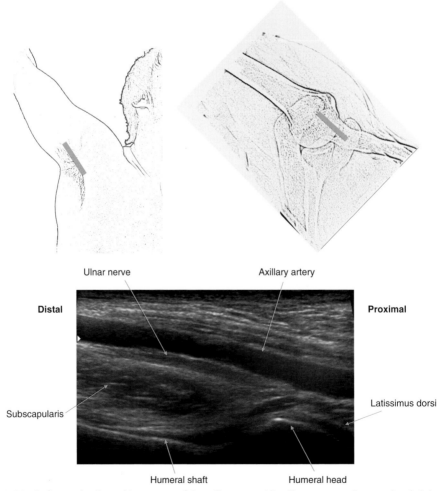

Fig. 1.20. Surface and radiographic anatomy of the axillary artery. LS, axilla, arm externally rotated and abducted.

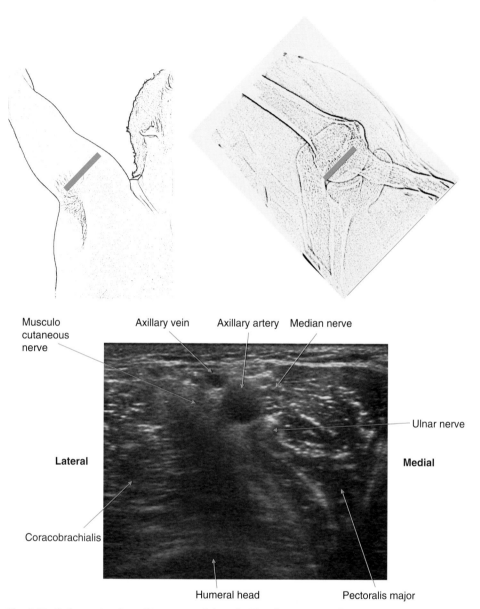

Fig. 1.21. Surface and radiographic anatomy of the axilla. TS, axilla, arm externally rotated and abducted.

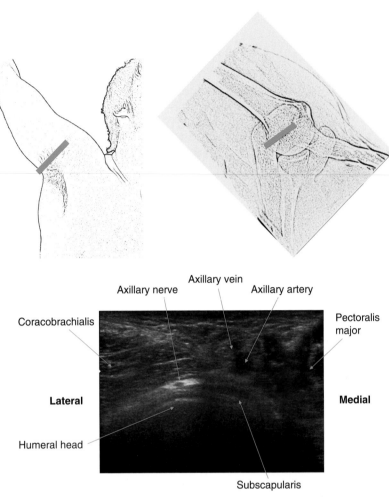

Fig. 1.22. Surface and radiographic anatomy of the axillary nerve. TS, axilla over humeral head and axillary artery.

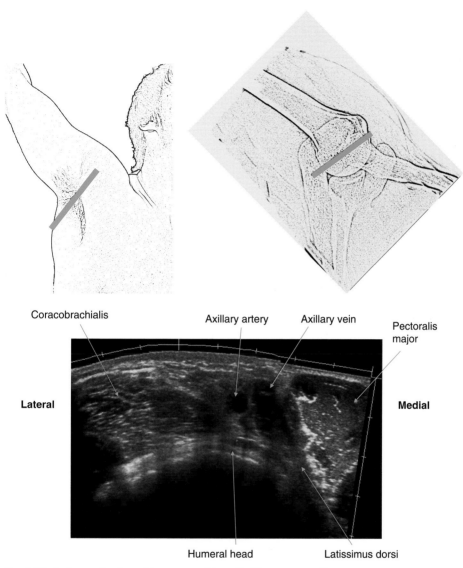

Fig. 1.23. Surface and radiographic anatomy of the axilla. TS, panorama axilla.

Upper limb

Shoulder

Acromioclavicular joint

Atypical synovial joint (articular surfaces lined with fibrocartilage), containing an incomplete articular disc. Surrounding capsule thickened superiorly to form acromioclavicular ligament.

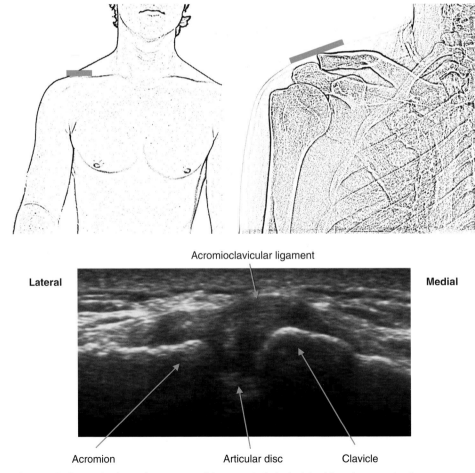

Acromioclavicular ligament

Lateral   Medial

Acromion   Articular disc   Clavicle

Fig. 2.1. Surface and radiographic anatomy of the acromioclavicular joint. LS, probe coronal, adjacent to superior aspect of joint. Arm adducted.

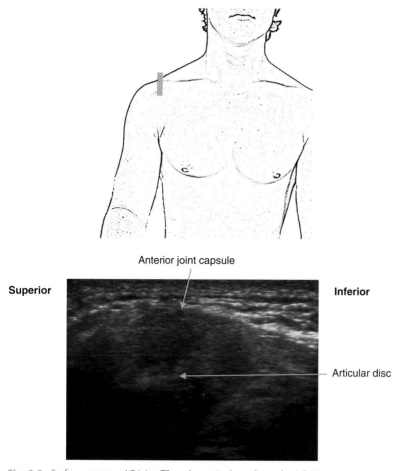

Superior

Inferior

Anterior joint capsule

Articular disc

Fig. 2.2. Surface anatomy AC joint. TS, probe sagittal, overlying the AC joint space.

Long head of biceps

It arises from the supraglenoid tubercle and adjacent glenoid labrum (biceps–labral complex) and traverses the glenohumeral joint surrounded by synovium to enter the bicipital groove. It is incompletely visible within the joint, but is reliably seen adjacent to the proximal humerus, where it is contained within its groove by the transverse ligament.

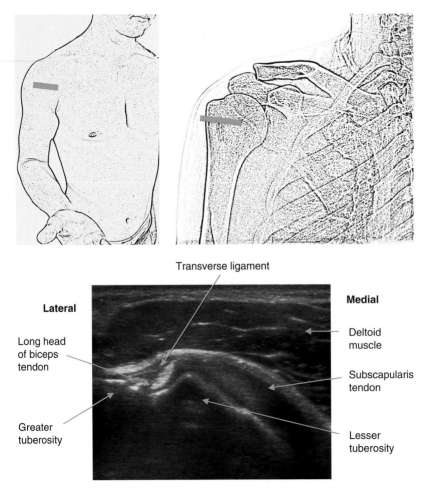

Fig. 2.3. Surface and radiographic anatomy of the long head of biceps tendon. TS, probe transverse across superior aspect of bicipital groove. Arm adducted, hand supinated. Examination of the rotator cuff is often conducted from behind the patient. Dynamic examination for subluxation of the tendon using internal and external rotation of the glenohumeral joint.

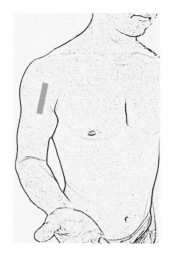

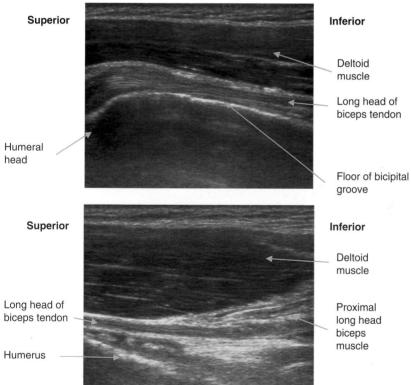

Superior Inferior

Deltoid
muscle

Long head of
biceps tendon

Humeral
head

Floor of bicipital
groove

Superior Inferior

Deltoid
muscle

Long head of
biceps tendon

Proximal
long head
biceps
muscle

Humerus

Fig. 2.4. Surface anatomy of the long head of biceps tendon. LS, probe longitudinal to long head of biceps tendon. Arm adducted, hand supinated.

Subscapularis

A multipennate muscle, originating from the costal surface of the scapula, whose tendon inserts into the lesser tuberosity of the humerus. It is separated from the shoulder joint by its bursa, which generally communicates with the joint cavity. Forms part of the posterior wall of axilla.

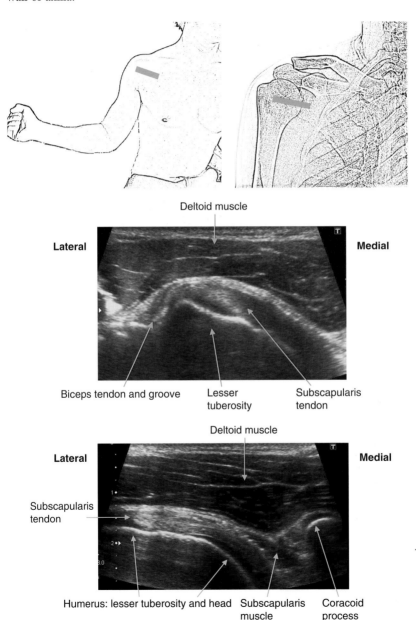

Fig. 2.5. Surface and radiographic anatomy of subscapularis tendon. LS, probe longitudinal to the subscapularis muscle (transverse to anterior shoulder), arm externally rotated with elbow kept against chest wall. Dynamic examination using internal and external rotation of the glenohumeral joint.

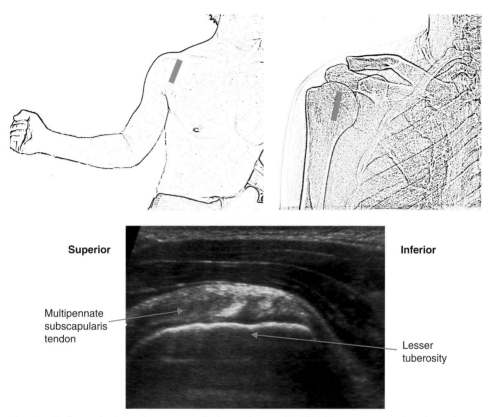

Fig. 2.6. Surface and radiographic anatomy of subscapularis tendon. TS, probe transverse to the subscapularis muscle (sagittal to anterior shoulder), arm externally rotated with elbow kept against chest wall.

Supraspinatus

Arises from the supraspinous fossa of the scapula and scapular spine. The tendon passes over the superior aspect of the shoulder joint to insert into the uppermost facet of the greater tuberosity of the humerus. The normal tendon shows a smooth, convex superior surface.

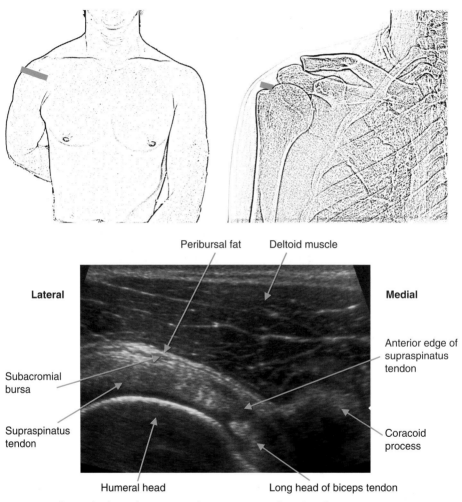

Fig. 2.7. Surface and radiographic anatomy of supraspinatus tendon. TS, probe transverse to supraspinatus tendon, with shoulder extended and internally rotated. Shoulder extension with internal rotation is required for clear visualization (back of hand in small of back, or 'hand-in wallet' position, elbow pointing posteriorly).

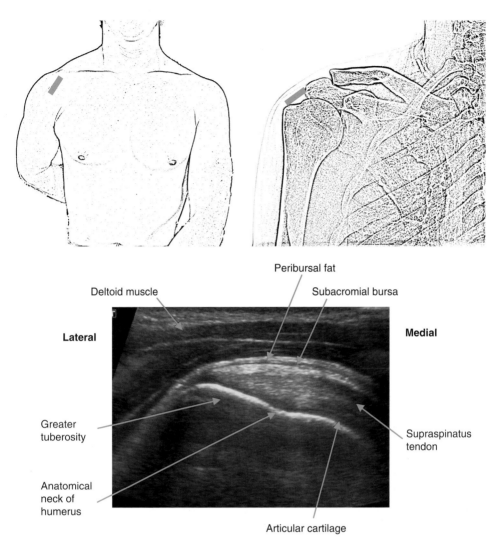

Fig. 2.8. Surface and radiographic anatomy of supraspinatus tendon. LS, probe longitudinal to supraspinatus tendon, with shoulder extended and internally rotated.

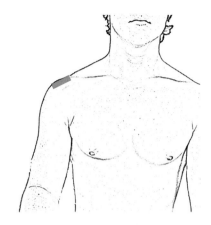

Adduction

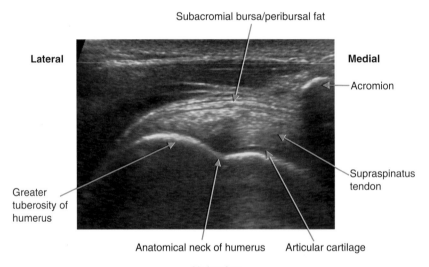

Subacromial bursa/peribursal fat

Lateral

Medial

Acromion

Greater
tuberosity of
humerus

Supraspinatus
tendon

Anatomical neck of humerus   Articular cartilage

Abduction

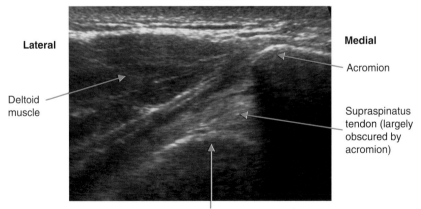

Lateral

Medial

Acromion

Deltoid
muscle

Supraspinatus
tendon (largely
obscured by
acromion)

Greater tuberosity of humerus

Fig. 2.8. (cont.) Dynamic assessment of supraspinatus can be useful in the further evaluation of impingement and cuff tears. Probe longitudinal over supraspinatus whilst abducting and adducting arm. This can be performed either from the front or back.

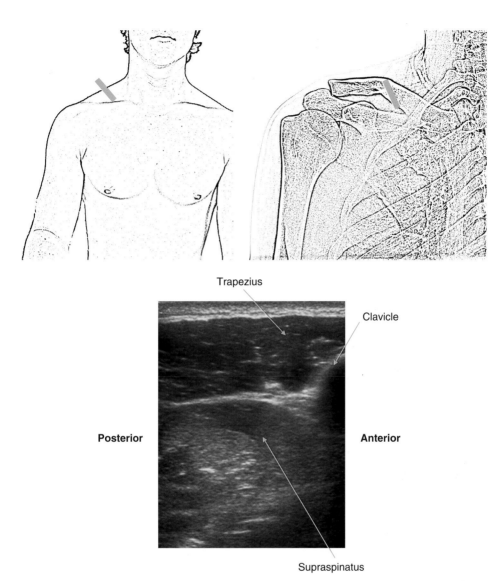

Fig. 2.9. Surface and radiographic anatomy of supraspinatus muscle. TS, probe medial to AC joint.

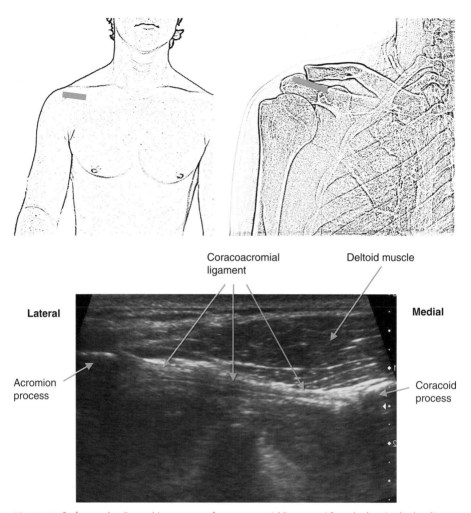

Fig. 2.10. Surface and radiographic anatomy of coracoacromial ligament. LS, probe longitudinal to ligament (transverse oblique to shoulder), with shoulder neutral. Dynamic assessment of the subacromial bursa relative to the ligament can also be useful for evaluation of impingement.

Infraspinatus

Arises from the infraspinous fossa on the posterior aspect of the scapula, inserting onto the middle facet of the greater tuberosity of the humerus. The muscular fibres often extend laterally for a greater distance, which occasionally allows distinction of this tendon from the adjacent supraspinatus and teres minor, which form a continuous cuff tendon.

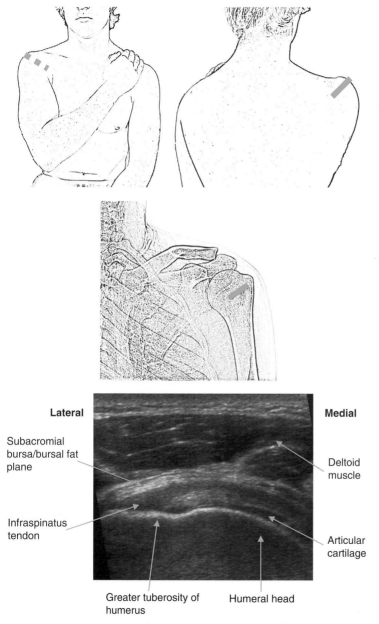

Fig. 2.11. Surface and radiographic anatomy of infraspinatus tendon. LS, probe longitudinal to infraspinatus tendon with shoulder flexed and adducted (hand on contralateral shoulder).

37

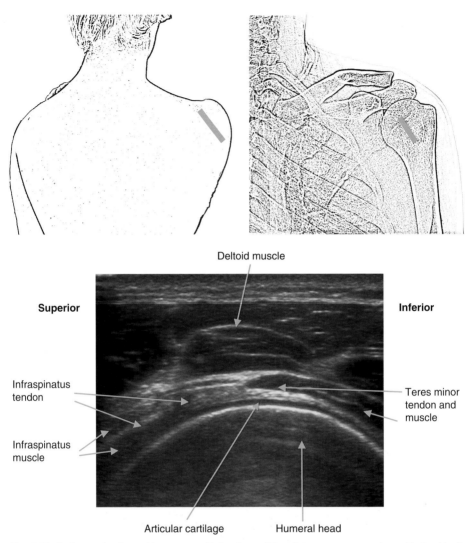

Fig. 2.12. Surface and radiographic anatomy of infraspinatus. TS, probe transverse to tendons with shoulder flexed and adducted (hand on contralateral shoulder).

Posterior joint

Visualizes infraspinatus and teres minor.

Teres minor

- Origin: upper two-thirds lateral border of scapula.
- Insertion: lower facet of greater tuberosity of humerus.

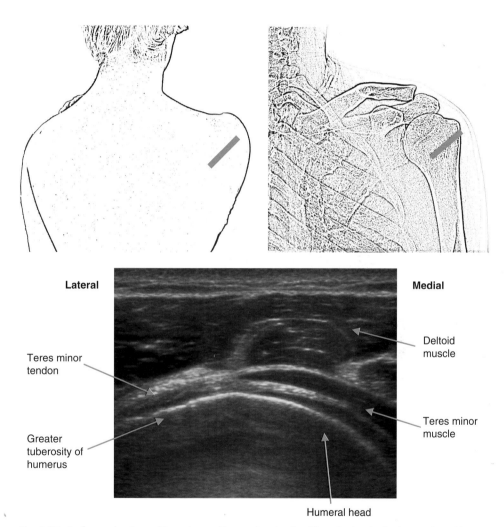

Fig. 2.13. Surface and radiographic anatomy of teres minor tendon. LS, probe longitudinal to tendon with shoulder flexed and adducted (hand on contralateral shoulder). Tendon inferior to infraspinatus.

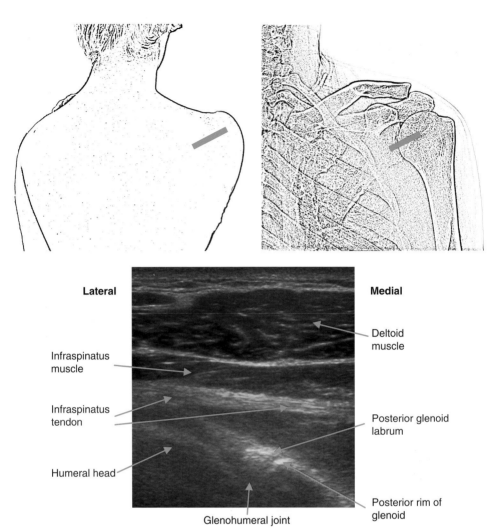

Lateral

Medial

Deltoid muscle

Infraspinatus muscle

Infraspinatus tendon

Posterior glenoid labrum

Humeral head

Glenohumeral joint

Posterior rim of glenoid

Fig. 2.14. Surface and radiographic anatomy of posterior shoulder. LS, probe longitudinal to posterior aspect of joint with shoulder flexed and adducted.

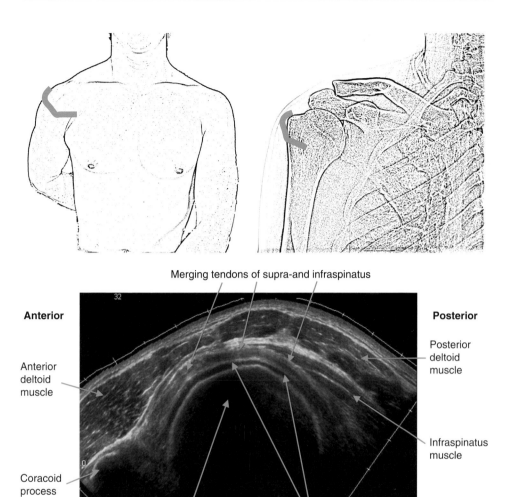

Anterior

Posterior

Merging tendons of supra-and infraspinatus

Posterior deltoid muscle

Anterior deltoid muscle

Infraspinatus muscle

Coracoid process

Humeral head

Humeral articular cartilage

Fig. 2.15. TS, panorama of rotator cuff.

Arm
Anterior

At the mid-point of the upper arm, biceps is the most superficial muscle group, with brachialis separating it from the humerus. The median nerve and brachial neurovascular bundle lie in a groove between biceps and triceps medially; the ulnar nerve/ulnar collateral artery lie adjacent to the median nerve posterior to the medial septum, and the radial neurovascular bundle, having passed posterior to the humerus in the spiral groove, pierces the lateral septum to enter the anterior compartment, eventually lying deep to brachioradialis.

Brachialis
- Origin: distal half of anterior humerus and medial intermuscular septum.
- Insertion: anterior surface of coronoid process of ulna.

Biceps
- Origin: short head from tip of coracoid process, long head from supraglenoid tubercle.
- Insertion: posterior part of radial tuberosity and the bicipital aponeurosis.

Coracobrachialis
- Origin: tip of coracoid process.
- Insertion: mid medial humerus.

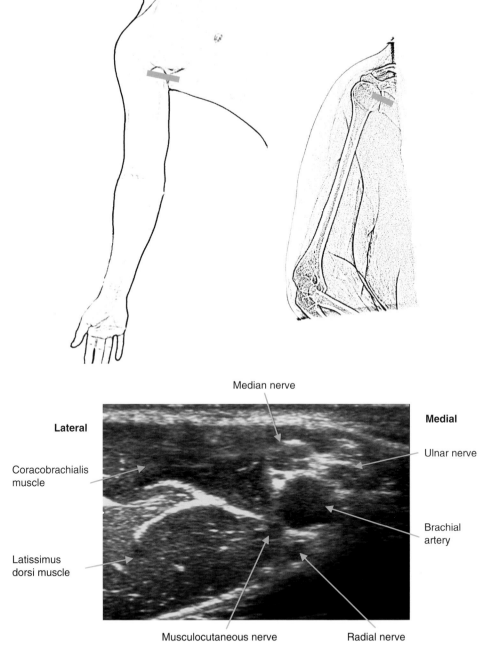

Fig. 2.16. Surface anatomy of upper arm. TS, probe transverse to anterior aspect of arm.

43

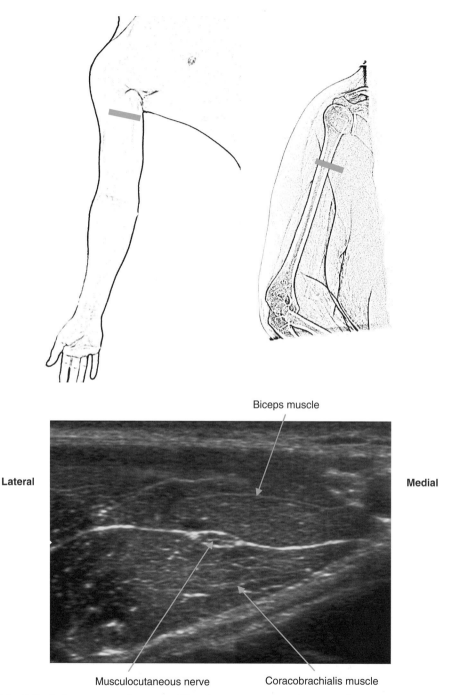

Fig. 2.17. Surface anatomy of upper arm. TS, probe transverse to anterior aspect of arm.

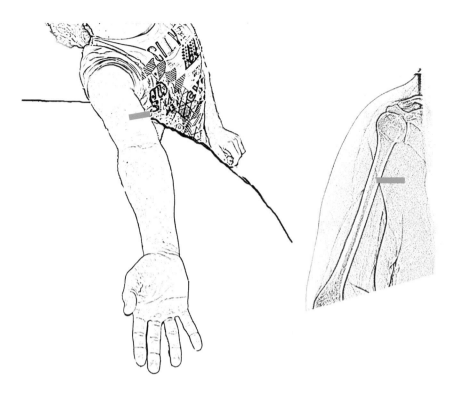

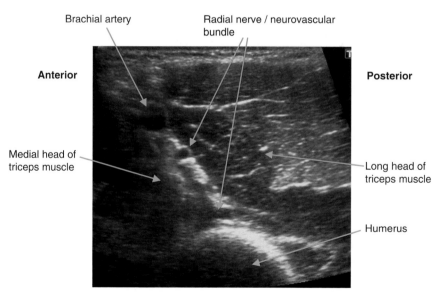

Brachial artery

Radial nerve / neurovascular bundle

Anterior

Posterior

Medial head of triceps muscle

Long head of triceps muscle

Humerus

Fig. 2.18. Surface anatomy medial arm. TS, probe transverse to medial aspect of arm, level of mid-humerus.

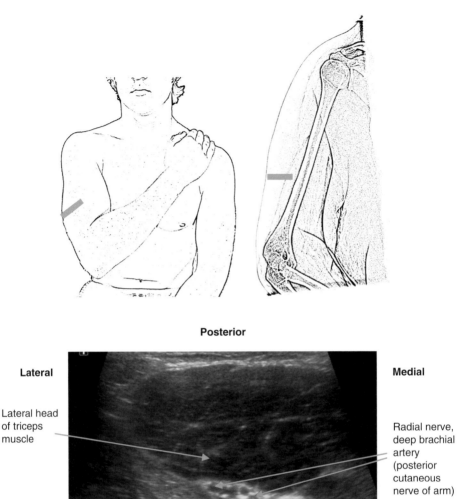

Posterior

Lateral

Medial

Lateral head
of triceps
muscle

Radial nerve,
deep brachial
artery
(posterior
cutaneous
nerve of arm)

Brachialis

Anterior   Humerus

Fig. 2.19. Surface anatomy radial nerve. TS, probe transverse to posterolateral aspect of humerus.

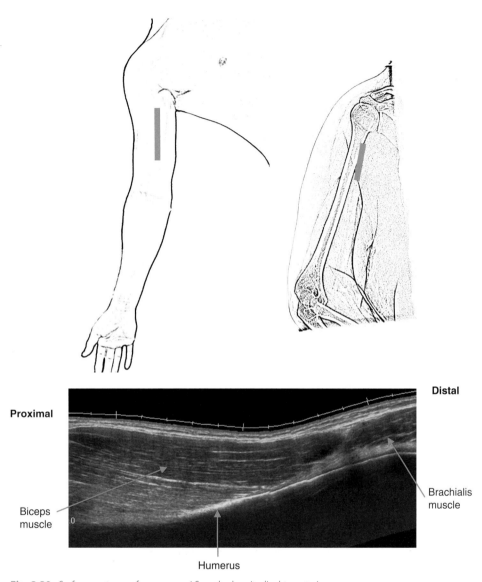

Proximal

Distal

Biceps
muscle

Brachialis
muscle

Humerus

Fig. 2.20. Surface anatomy of upper arm. LS, probe longitudinal to anterior arm.

Posterior arm
Triceps

- Origin: long head from the infraglenoid tubercle, lateral head from upper border of radial groove of humerus, medial head from posterior surface of humerus and intermuscular septum.
- Insertion: olecranon process of ulna.

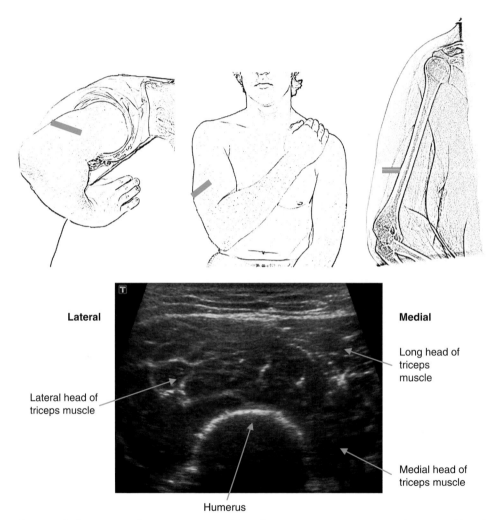

Lateral

Medial

Long head of triceps muscle

Lateral head of triceps muscle

Medial head of triceps muscle

Humerus

Fig. 2.21. Surface anatomy of arm, posterior aspect. TS, probe transverse to posterior aspect of arm, arm adducted and elbow flexed (holding opposite shoulder) or elbow flexed to expose posterior aspect.

Elbow

Lateral elbow

Important anatomical structures in this region of the elbow include the common extensor origin (CEO). This comprises the fused tendons of extensor carpi radialis brevis, extensor digitorum, extensor digiti minimi and extensor carpi ulnaris, which attach anteriorly to the lateral epicondyle of the humerus.

The superficial group of posterior and lateral forearm muscles are brachioradialis and extensor carpi radialis longus. They originate proximal to the CEO, from the lateral supracondylar ridge of the humerus.

Brachioradialis
- Origin: lateral supracondylar ridge of humerus.
- Insertion: lateral aspect distal radius.

Extensor carpi radialis longus
- Origin: lateral supracondylar ridge of humerus.
- Insertion: dorsal surface base of index finger metacarpal.

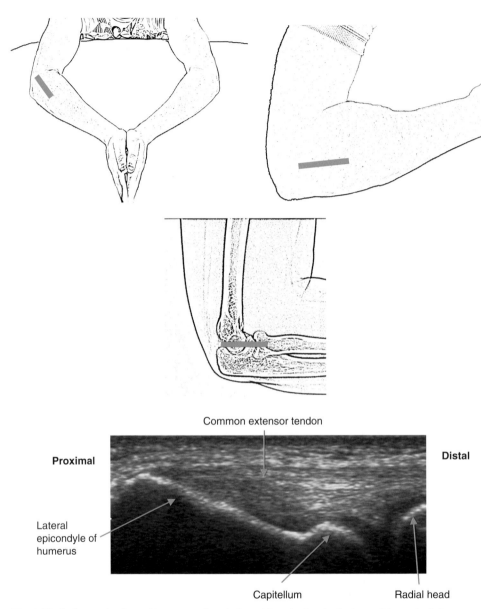

Common extensor tendon

Proximal

Distal

Lateral
epicondyle of
humerus

Capitellum

Radial head

Fig. 2.22. Surface and radiographic anatomy lateral elbow. LS, probe longitudinal to radial aspect of elbow, hand in mid-supinated position. Comparison with the contralateral side facilitated by 'praying' position.

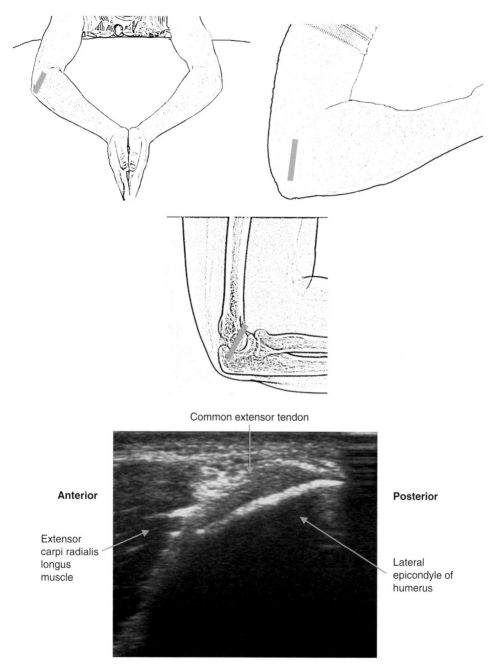

Common extensor tendon

Anterior

Posterior

Extensor
carpi radialis
longus
muscle

Lateral
epicondyle of
humerus

Fig. 2.23. Surface and radiographic anatomy lateral elbow. TS, probe transverse to radial aspect of elbow, hand in mid-supinated position.

The radiocapitellar joint and annular ligament
Annular ligament
Encircles head of radius, attached to the anterior and posterior borders of the radial notch of the ulna.

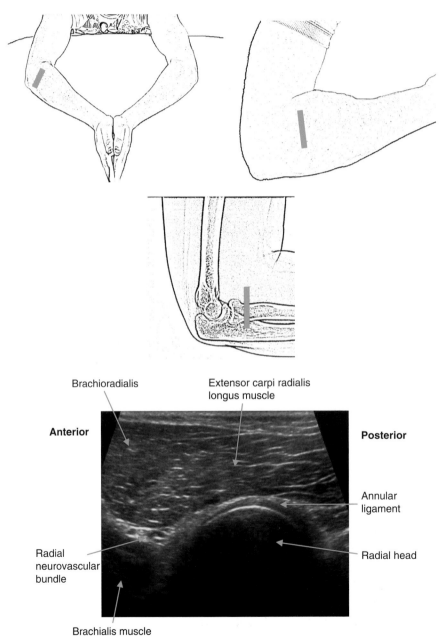

Fig. 2.24. Surface and radiographic anatomy lateral elbow. TS, probe transverse to elbow, longitudinal to annular ligament at level of radial head and slightly distal to common extensor tendon origin.

Anterior elbow

Visualizes the anterior aspect of the elbow joint, neurovascular structures and biceps tendon.

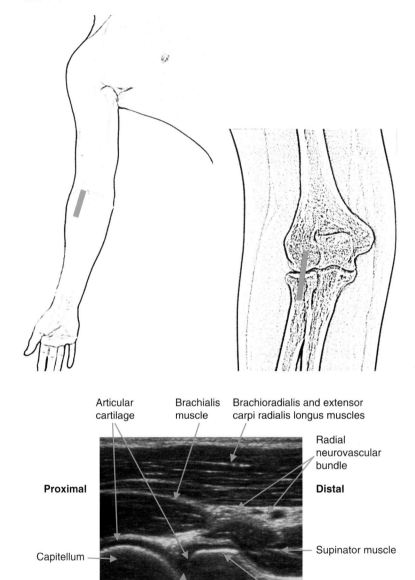

Fig. 2.25. Surface anatomy anterolateral elbow. LS, probe longitudinal, elbow extended, hand supinated.

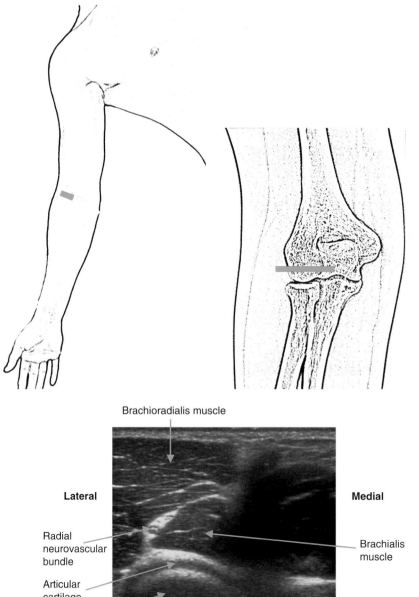

Brachioradialis muscle

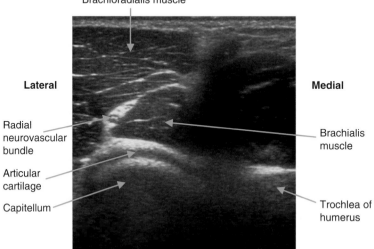

Lateral

Radial
neurovascular
bundle

Articular
cartilage

Capitellum

Medial

Brachialis
muscle

Trochlea of
humerus

Fig. 2.26. Surface and radiographic anatomy anterolateral elbow. TS, probe transverse, elbow extended, hand supinated.

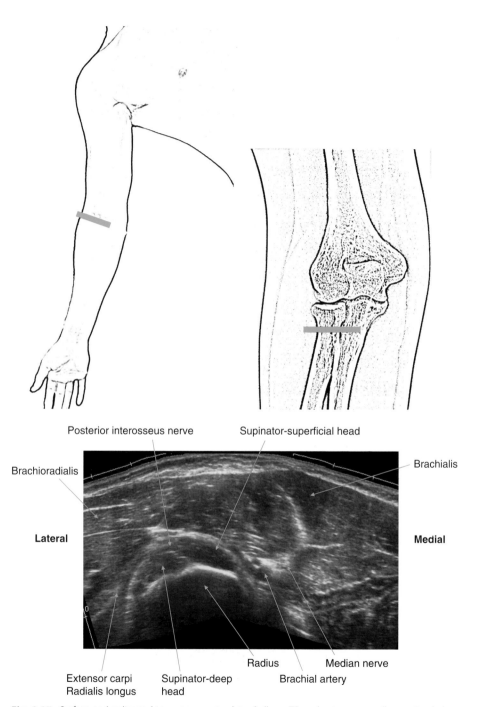

Fig. 2.27. Surface and radiographic anatomy anterolateral elbow. TS, probe transverse, elbow extended, hand supinated.

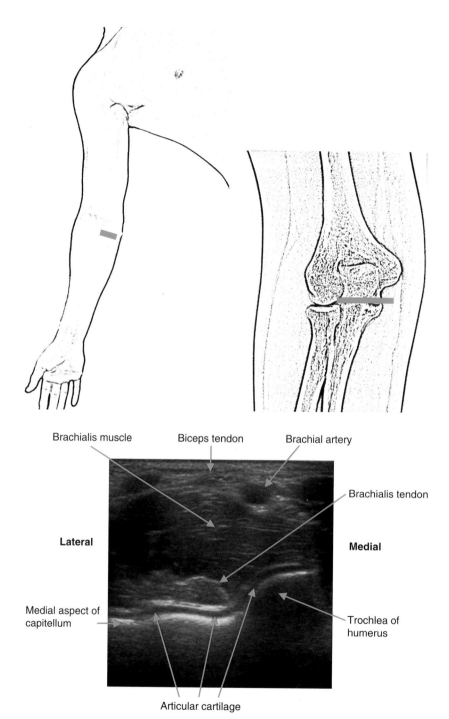

Fig. 2.28. Surface and radiographic anatomy anteromedial elbow. TS, probe transverse to anterior elbow, elbow extended, hand supinated.

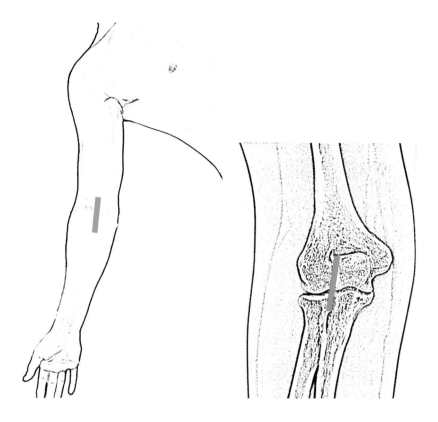

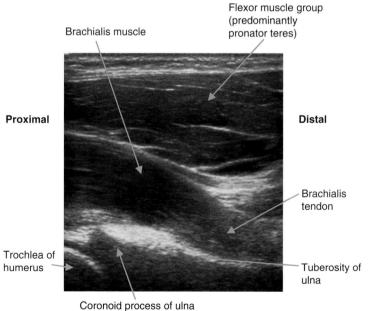

Brachialis muscle

Flexor muscle group
(predominantly
pronator teres)

Proximal

Distal

Brachialis
tendon

Trochlea of
humerus

Tuberosity of
ulna

Coronoid process of ulna

Fig. 2.29. Surface and radiographic anatomy anterior elbow. LS, probe longitudinal to anteromedial elbow, elbow extended.

Biceps tendon

It inserts onto the tuberosity of the radius, and a bursa separates bone and tendon just proximal to the insertion. A further insertion is via the bicipital aponeurosis into the deep fascia on the ulnar aspect of the forearm and posterior subcutaneous border of the ulna.

It can be difficult to demonstrate the tendon due to anisotropy as it travels deeper to its insertion.

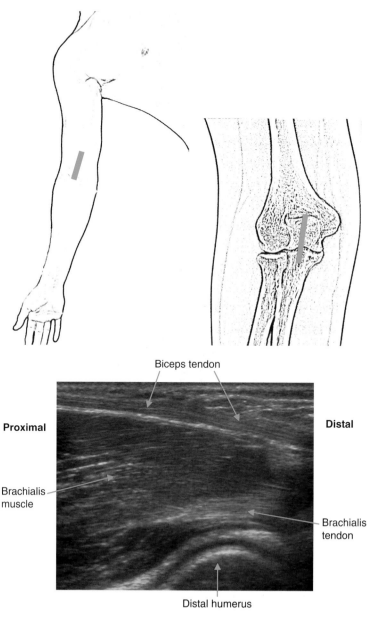

Biceps tendon

Proximal

Distal

Brachialis muscle

Brachialis tendon

Distal humerus

Fig. 2.30. Surface and radiographic anatomy distal biceps tendon. LS, probe longitudinal, slightly oblique to long axis of upper limb, elbow extended.

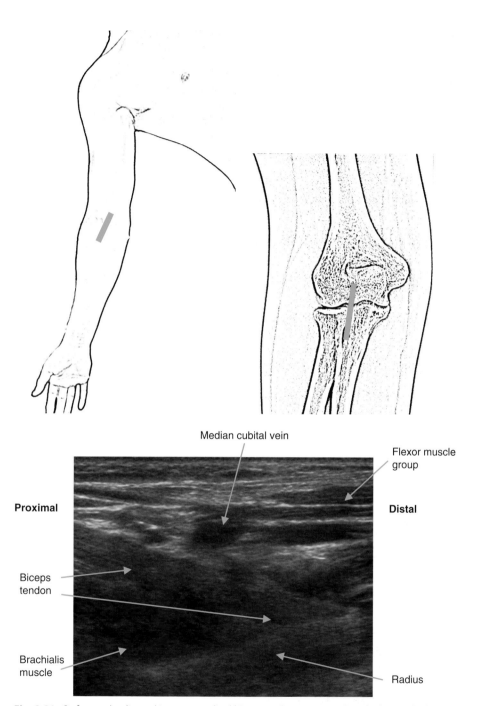

Median cubital vein

Flexor muscle group

Proximal

Distal

Biceps tendon

Brachialis muscle

Radius

Fig. 2.31. Surface and radiographic anatomy, distal biceps tendon insertion. LS, probe longitudinal, elbow extended (slight flexion may aid visualization of distal tendon).

Medial elbow

Pathologically and anatomically important structures here include the common flexor origin (CFO), ulnar collateral ligament and medial aspect of the elbow joint.

The CFO is situated anteriorly on the medial epicondyle of the humerus, and gives origin to the superficial muscle group of pronator teres, flexor carpi radialis, flexor digitorum superficialis, palmaris longus and flexor carpi ulnaris. These muscles form the medial border of the cubital fossa.

The deep forearm muscles include, flexor pollicis longus, flexor digitorum profundus and pronator quadratus.

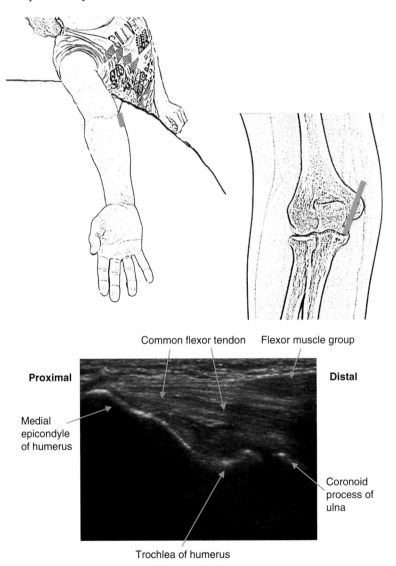

Fig. 2.32. Surface and radiographic anatomy medial elbow. LS, probe longitudinal to common flexor tendon origin, access to which is improved if the patient leans to the lateral side.

Ulnar collateral ligament (UCL)

This triangular ligament has three parts.

- The strongest is the anterior band, which can be seen deep to the CFO, running from the medial epicondyle of the humerus to the coronoid process of the ulna (the 'sublime' tubercle).
- The posterior band runs posteriorly from the sublime tubercle to the olecranon.
- The transverse band spans anterior and posterior.

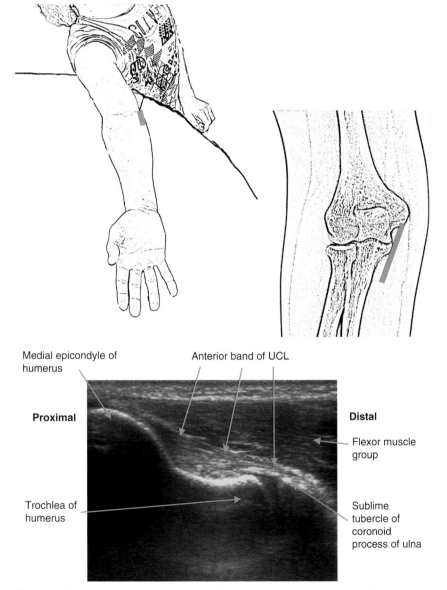

Medial epicondyle of humerus

Anterior band of UCL

Proximal

Distal

Flexor muscle group

Trochlea of humerus

Sublime tubercle of coronoid process of ulna

Fig. 2.33. Surface and radiographic anatomy of the anterior band of ulnar collateral ligament. LS, probe longitudinal to medial elbow (similar position to CFO).

Posterior elbow

The triceps tendon attaches to the olecranon of the ulna.

The ulnar nerve can be seen in a groove posterior to medial humeral epicondyle.

Examination of the posterior elbow is facilitated by placing the joint in one of two positions.

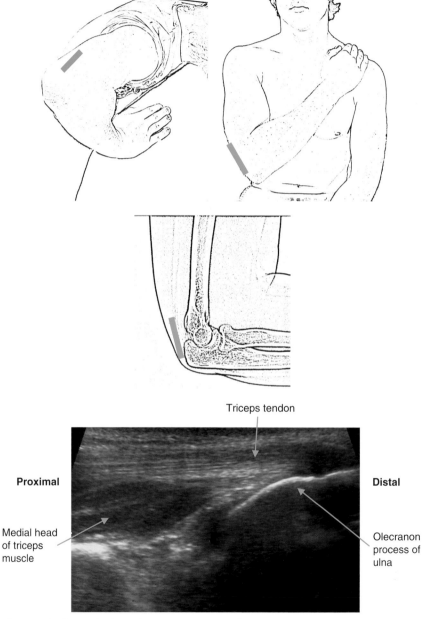

Triceps tendon

Proximal

Distal

Medial head of triceps muscle

Olecranon process of ulna

Fig. 2.34. Surface and radiographic anatomy posterior elbow. LS, probe longitudinal to posterior elbow, patient in 'crab' position or arm adducted, holding contralateral shoulder.

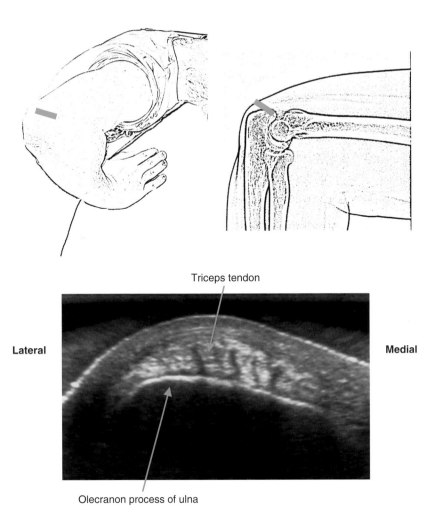

Triceps tendon

Lateral

Medial

Olecranon process of ulna

Fig. 2.35. Surface and radiographic anatomy posterior elbow. TS, probe transverse to posterior elbow, patient in 'crab' position.

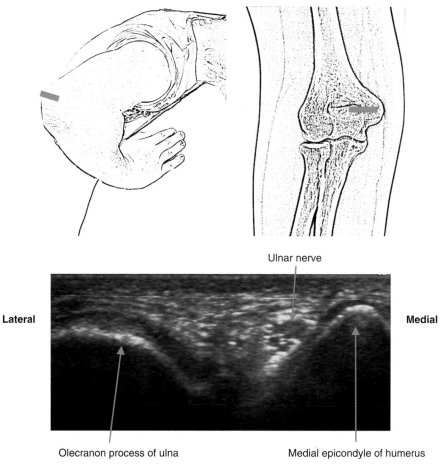

Ulnar nerve

Lateral

Medial

Olecranon process of ulna

Medial epicondyle of humerus

Fig. 2.36. Surface and radiographic anatomy ulnar nerve. TS, probe transverse to posteromedial elbow. Ulnar nerve in the ulnar groove.

Forearm
Anterior

The superficial muscles arise from the common flexor origin. They are from lateral to medial: pronator teres, flexor carpi radialis, palmaris longus, flexor digitorum superficialis, flexor carpi ulnaris.

The deep muscles include flexor pollicis longus, flexor digitorum profundus and pronator quadratus.

The course of the median nerve can be followed from elbow to wrist. It emerges from the cubital fossa, where it is medial to the brachial artery. It passes between the heads of pronator teres, and descends between flexors superficialis and profundus. At the wrist, it lies deep to the flexor retinaculum, between flexor carpi radialis and flexor digitorum superficialis.

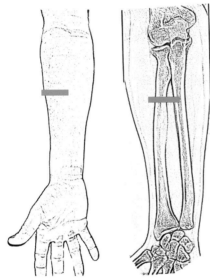

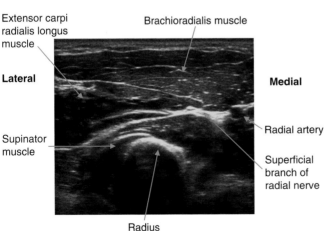

Fig. 2.37. Surface and radiographic anatomy proximal forearm. TS, probe transverse on radial aspect forearm (junction of proximal and middle thirds).

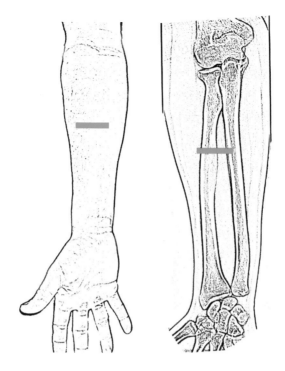

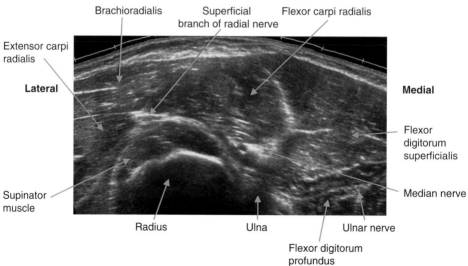

Extensor carpi radialis

Brachioradialis

Superficial branch of radial nerve

Flexor carpi radialis

Lateral

Medial

Supinator muscle

Flexor digitorum superficialis

Median nerve

Radius

Ulna

Ulnar nerve

Flexor digitorum profundus

Fig. 2.38. Surface and radiographic anatomy mid forearm. TS panorama, probe transverse to anterior forearm.

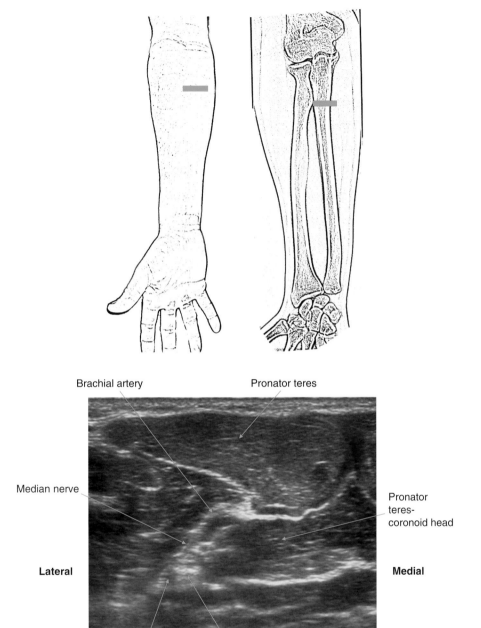

Fig. 2.39. Surface and radiographic anatomy proximal forearm. TS, probe transverse on ulnar aspect forearm (junction of proximal and middle thirds).

Distal forearm

Movement of the fingers helps to distinguish the median nerve from flexor tendons. It can also be followed proximally to the elbow, and no muscle belly appears. Its appearances are otherwise often quite similar to a tendon.

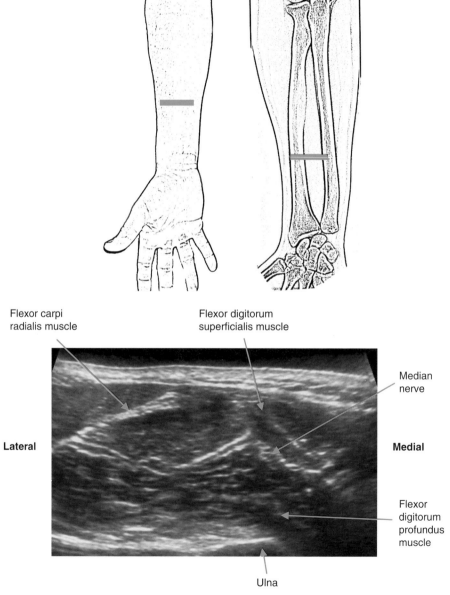

Flexor carpi radialis muscle

Flexor digitorum superficialis muscle

Median nerve

Lateral

Medial

Flexor digitorum profundus muscle

Ulna

Fig. 2.40. Surface and radiographic anatomy distal forearm. TS, probe transverse to distal anterior forearm.

Posterior forearm

The superficial muscle group arises from the lateral supracondylar ridge of the humerus, and includes brachioradialis and extensor carpi radialis longus.

The posterior muscle group arises from the common extensor origin, and comprises extensor carpi radialis brevis, extensor digitorum, extensor digiti minimi and extensor carpi ulnaris.

The deep muscle group includes supinator, abductor pollicis longus, extensor pollicis brevis, extensor pollicis longus and extensor indicis.

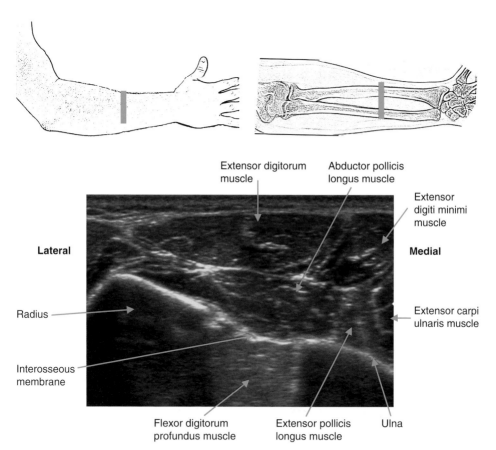

Fig. 2.41. Surface and radiographic anatomy posterior forearm. TS, probe transverse to posterior forearm.

Wrist

Anterior

Carpal tunnel

The roof of the tunnel is formed by the flexor retinaculum, which is attached on the radial side to the tuberosity of the scaphoid and ridge of the trapezium, and on the ulnar side to the pisiform and hook of the hamate. The carpal bones form the floor.

From lateral to medial, the major contents are: flexor pollicis longus (deep to median nerve), flexor digitorum superficialis and profundus. Palmaris longus, if present, passes superficial to the retinaculum.

The ulnar nerve lies on the retinaculum alongside the pisiform, medial to the ulnar artery. Both are covered by a superficial part of the retinaculum (the volar (palmar) carpal ligament), forming Guyon's canal. The abductor digiti minimi muscle belly varies in size and can cause ulnar nerve symptoms.

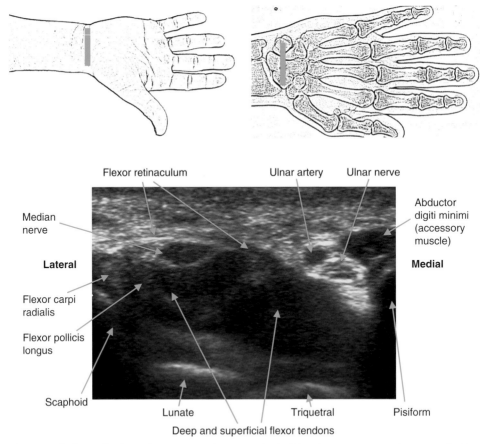

Fig. 2.42. Surface and radiographic anatomy volar aspect of wrist. TS, probe transverse to volar aspect of wrist, level of proximal carpal tunnel.

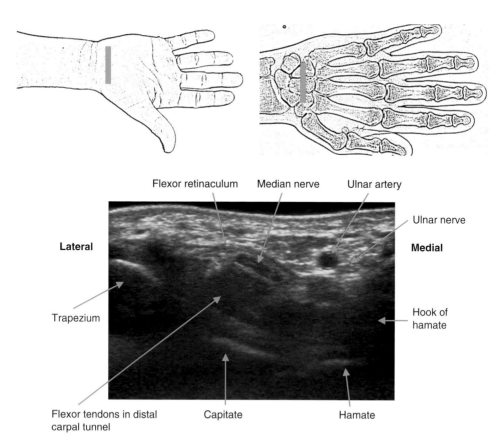

Flexor retinaculum   Median nerve   Ulnar artery

Ulnar nerve

Lateral   **Medial**

Trapezium

Hook of hamate

Flexor tendons in distal   Capitate   Hamate
carpal tunnel

Fig. 2.43. Surface and radiographic anatomy volar aspect of wrist. TS, probe transverse to volar aspect of wrist, level of distal carpal tunnel.

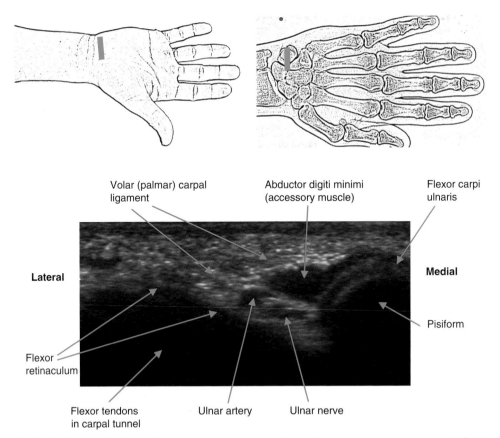

Fig. 2.44. Surface and radiographic anatomy volar ulnar aspect of wrist. TS, probe transverse to volar aspect of wrist at ulnar aspect of carpal tunnel.

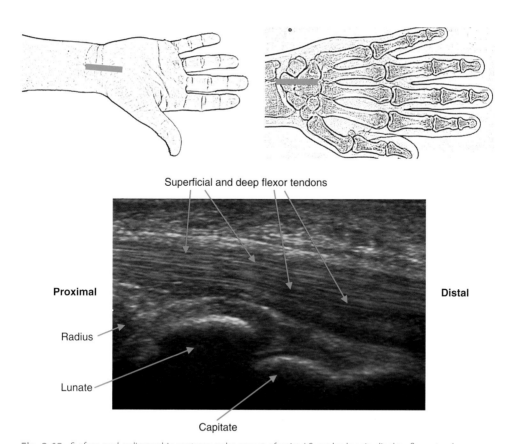

Superficial and deep flexor tendons

Proximal

Distal

Radius

Lunate

Capitate

Fig. 2.45. Surface and radiographic anatomy volar aspect of wrist. LS, probe longitudinal to flexor tendons.

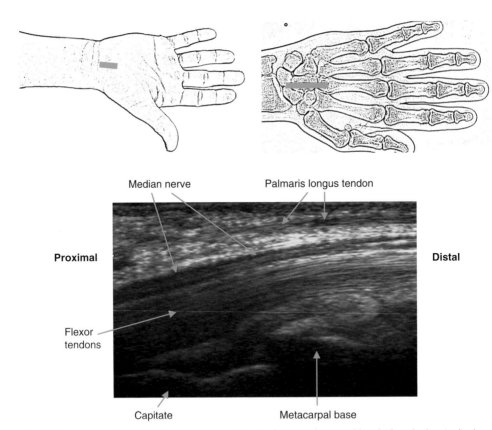

Fig. 2.46. Surface and radiographic anatomy volar aspect of wrist and proximal hand. LS, probe longitudinal to flexor tendons.

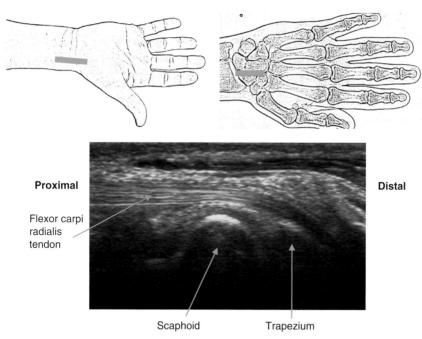

Proximal

Distal

Flexor carpi
radialis
tendon

Scaphoid   Trapezium

Fig. 2.47. Surface and radiographic anatomy volar radial aspect of wrist. LS, probe longitudinal to flexor carpi radialis tendon.

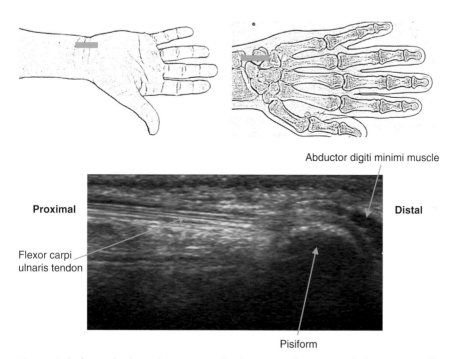

Abductor digiti minimi muscle

Proximal

Distal

Flexor carpi
ulnaris tendon

Pisiform

Fig. 2.48. Surface and radiographic anatomy volar ulnar aspect of wrist. LS, probe longitudinal to flexor carpi ulnaris tendon.

Lateral

Anatomical snuffbox

Proximally, the snuffbox is demarcated by the radial styloid, and distally by the base of the thumb metacarpal. Its radial boundary is formed by two tendons (extensor pollicis brevis and abductor pollicis longus) and on the ulnar aspect by extensor pollicis longus. The floor of the snuffbox is formed by the scaphoid proximally and the trapezium distally. It contains the radial artery and cephalic vein.

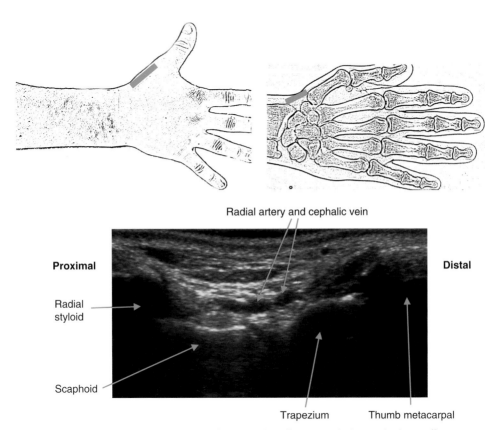

Fig. 2.49. Surface and radiographic anatomy of anatomical snuffbox. LS, probe longitudinal to snuffbox, radial aspect of wrist. Ulnar deviation of the wrist with extension of the thumb.

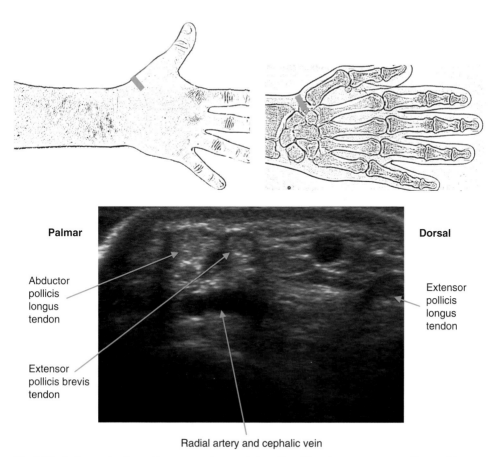

Palmar

Dorsal

Abductor
pollicis
longus
tendon

Extensor
pollicis
longus
tendon

Extensor
pollicis brevis
tendon

Radial artery and cephalic vein

Fig. 2.50. Surface and radiographic anatomy of anatomical snuffbox. TS, probe transverse to snuffbox, radial aspect of wrist. Ulnar deviation of the wrist with extension of the thumb.

Thumb carpometacarpal joint

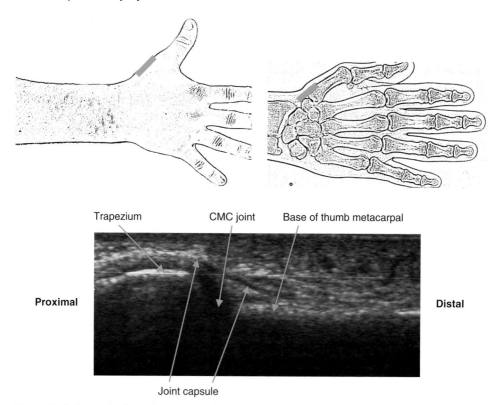

Trapezium   CMC joint   Base of thumb metacarpal

Proximal   Distal

Joint capsule

Fig. 2.51. Surface and radiographic anatomy of thumb carpometacarpal joint. LS, probe longitudinal to thumb carpometacarpal joint.

Posterior

At the level of the distal radius the extensor tendons occupy six distinct compartments.

I: abductor pollicis longus (volar) and extensor pollicis brevis.

II: extensor carpi radialis longus (radial) and brevis.

III: extensor pollicis longus (subsequently passes superficial to the extensor carpi radialis tendons to form the posterior border of the anatomical snuffbox).

IV: extensor indicis (radial) and extensor digitorum.

V: extensor digiti minimi.

VI: extensor carpi ulnaris.

The dorsal tubercle of the radius (Lister's tubercle) is a useful landmark, separating extensor compartments (ECs) II and III.

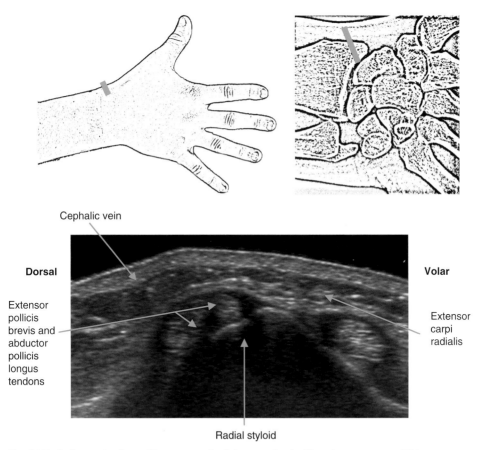

Cephalic vein

Dorsal

Volar

Extensor pollicis brevis and abductor pollicis longus tendons

Extensor carpi radialis

Radial styloid

Fig. 2.52. Surface and radiographic anatomy of radial aspect of wrist. TS, probe transverse to EC I.

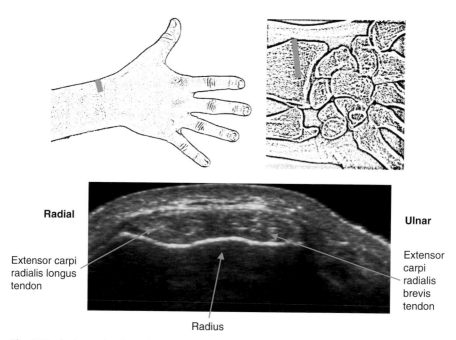

Radial

Ulnar

Extensor carpi
radialis longus
tendon

Extensor
carpi
radialis
brevis
tendon

Radius

Fig. 2.53. Surface and radiographic anatomy of radial aspect of wrist. TS, probe transverse to EC II.

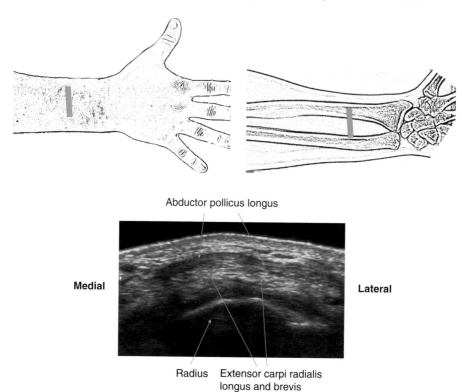

Abductor pollicus longus

Medial

Lateral

Radius   Extensor carpi radialis
longus and brevis

Fig. 2.54. Surface and radiographic anatomy of radial aspect of wrist at crossover of first and second extensor compartments. TS, probe transverse over distal radius.

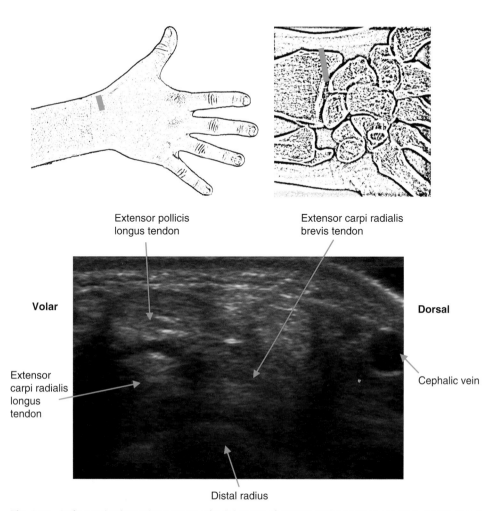

Fig. 2.55. Surface and radiographic anatomy of radial aspect of wrist. TS, probe transverse to EC II, distal to Lister's tubercle.

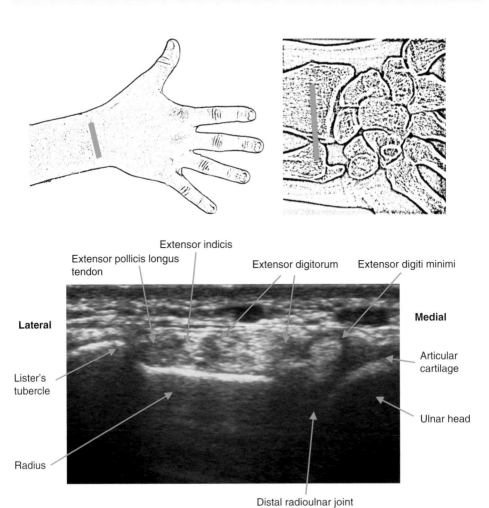

Fig. 2.56. Surface and radiographic anatomy of dorsal aspect of wrist. TS, probe transverse to wrist at level of Lister's tubercle.

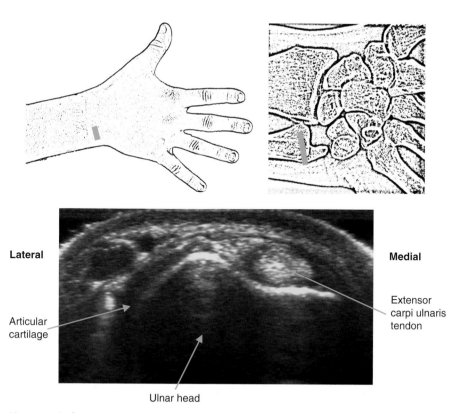

Lateral

Medial

Articular
cartilage

Extensor
carpi ulnaris
tendon

Ulnar head

Fig. 2.57. Surface and radiographic anatomy of dorsal aspect of wrist. TS, probe transverse to EC VI.

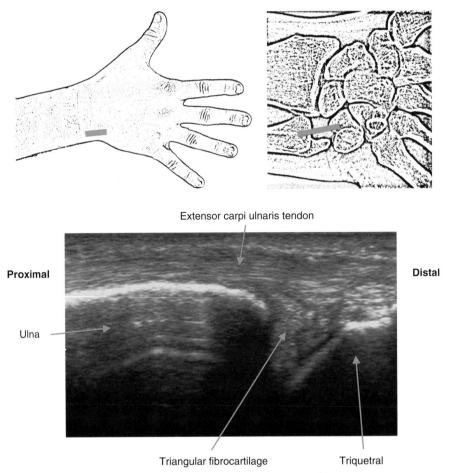

Extensor carpi ulnaris tendon

Proximal

Distal

Ulna

Triangular fibrocartilage

Triquetral

Fig. 2.58. Surface and radiographic anatomy of dorsal aspect of wrist. LS, probe longitudinal to EC VI.

Interosseous scapholunate ligament

The dorsal aspect of this ligament is seen as a high reflectivity linear structure in the scapholunate space.

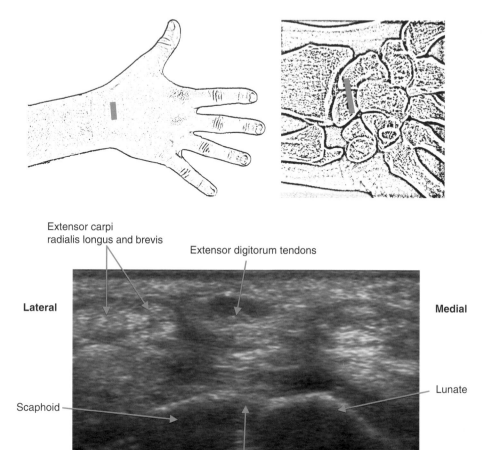

Fig. 2.59. Surface and radiographic anatomy of interosseous scapholunate ligament. TS, probe transverse to dorsal aspect of wrist, level of proximal carpal row.

Hand
Palm
Palmar spaces

The palm is divided into three spaces by two septa passing from the palmar aponeurosis to the thumb and little finger metacarpals. The lateral space contains thenar muscles; the medial contains hypothenar muscles, and the central contains long flexor tendons, lumbricals, the superficial and deep palmar arches and median nerve.

Central palmar space

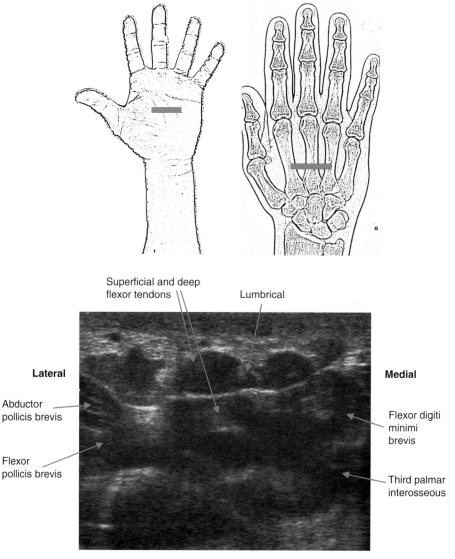

Fig. 2.60. Surface and radiographic anatomy central palm. TS, probe transverse to flexor tendons in proximal palm.

Medial (hypothenar) and lateral (thenar) palmar spaces

- The muscles in the hypothenar eminence are abductor digiti minimi, opponens digiti minimi and flexor digiti minimi brevis.
- The muscles in the thenar eminence are abductor pollicis brevis, opponens pollicis and flexor pollicis brevis.

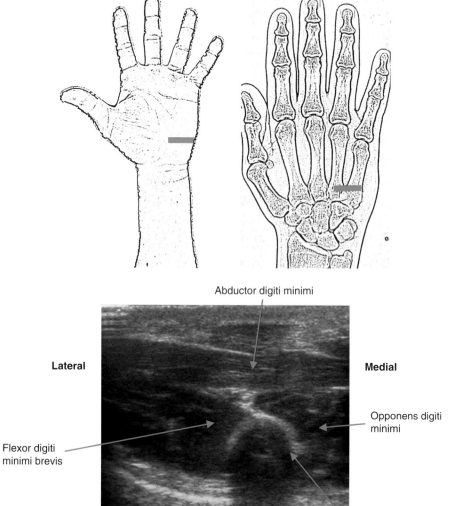

Fig. 2.61. Surface and radiographic anatomy hypothenar eminence. TS, probe transverse on hypothenar eminence.

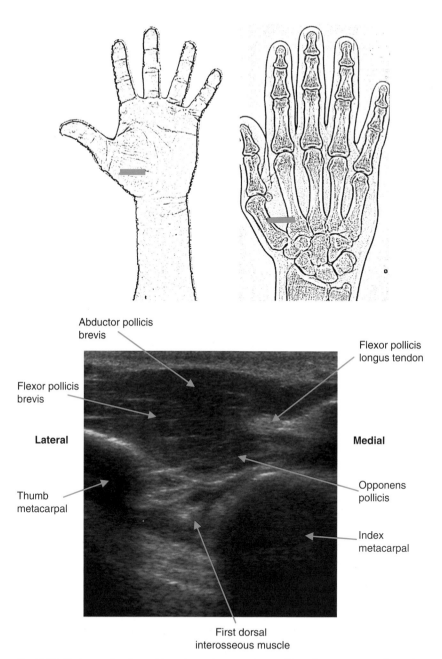

Fig. 2.62. Surface and radiographic anatomy thenar eminence. TS, probe transverse on hypo thenar eminence.

Flexor tendons

The superficial flexor tendons pass deep to the flexor retinaculum at the wrist. In the palm they are contained within a common flexor sheath, superficial to the profundus tendons. This relationship continues in the common synovial sheath of the finger. The superficialis tendon splits at the level of the proximal phalanx, and is pierced by the profundus tendon, which is therefore the most superficial tendon at the distal part of the proximal phalanx. The superficial tendon inserts onto the sides of the palmar surface of the middle phalanx, and the deep tendon continues to the base of the distal phalanx.

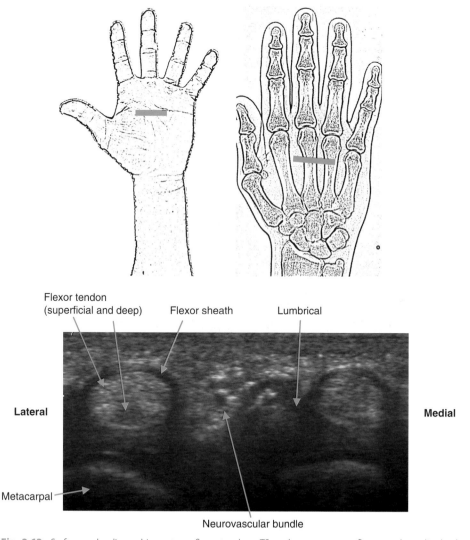

Fig. 2.63. Surface and radiographic anatomy flexor tendons. TS, probe transverse to flexor tendons, distal palm.

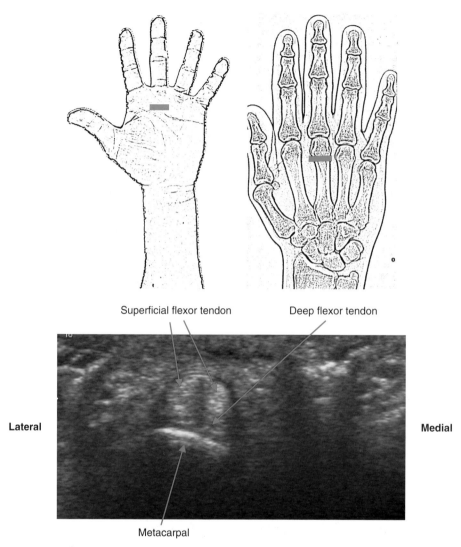

Fig. 2.64. Surface and radiographic anatomy flexor tendons. TS, probe transverse over metacarpal neck.

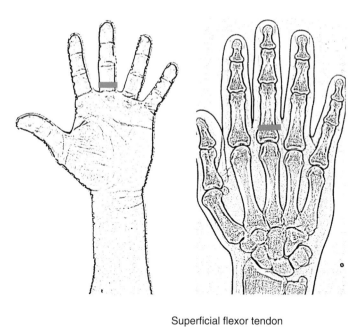

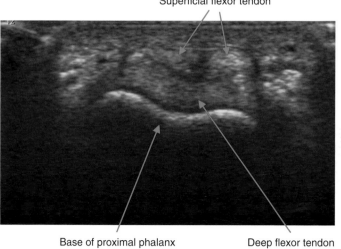

Superficial flexor tendon

Lateral

Medial

Base of proximal phalanx

Deep flexor tendon

Fig. 2.65. Surface and radiographic anatomy flexor tendons. TS, probe transverse over base of proximal phalanx.

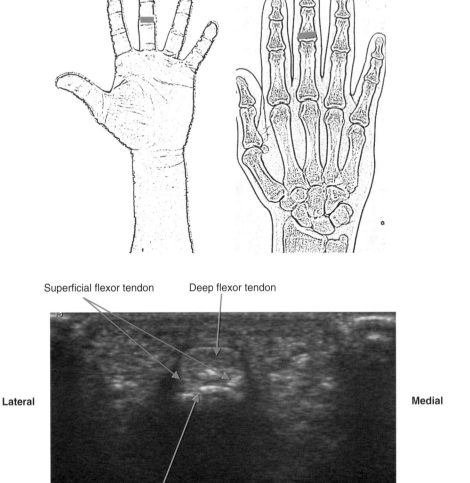

Fig. 2.66. Surface and radiographic anatomy flexor tendons. TS, probe transverse over base of middle phalanx.

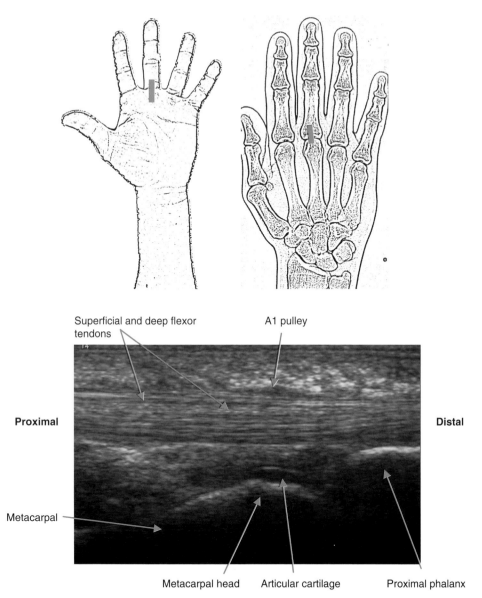

Fig. 2.67. Surface and radiographic anatomy flexor tendons. LS, probe longitudinal over metacarpophalangeal joint. Dynamic assessment with finger flexion and extension.

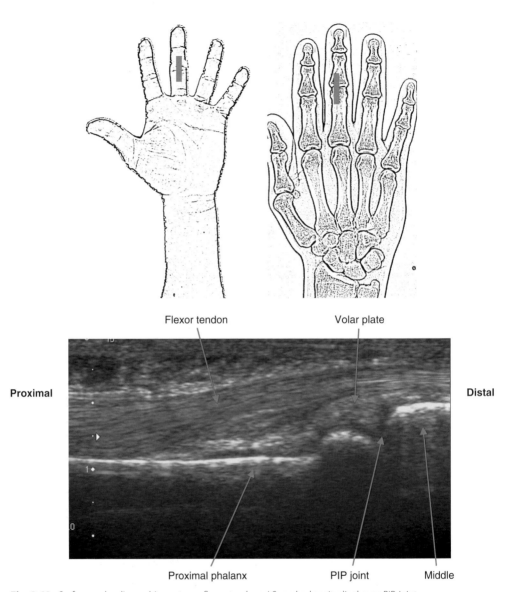

Fig. 2.68. Surface and radiographic anatomy flexor tendons. LS, probe longitudinal over PIP joint.

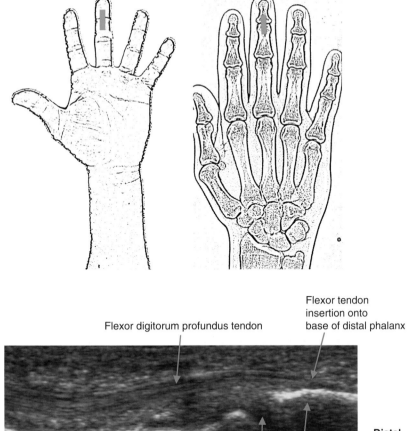

Flexor tendon insertion onto base of distal phalanx

Flexor digitorum profundus tendon

Proximal

Distal

Middle phalanx   DIP joint   Distal phalanx

Fig. 2.69. Surface and radiographic anatomy flexor tendons. LS, probe longitudinal over DIP joint.

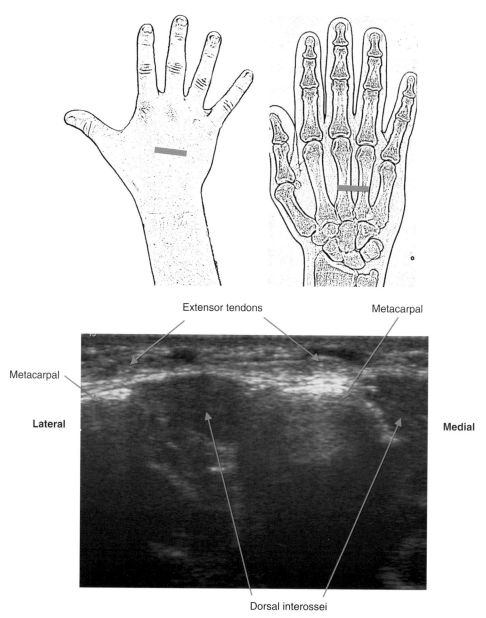

Extensor tendons   Metacarpal

Metacarpal

Lateral   Medial

Dorsal interossei

Fig. 2.70. Surface and radiographic anatomy extensor tendons. TS, probe transverse over dorsum of hand, proximal metacarpal level.

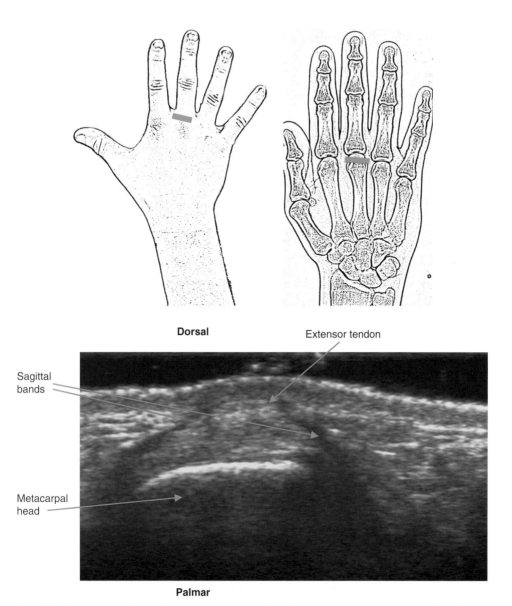

Dorsal

Extensor tendon

Sagittal bands

Metacarpal head

Palmar

Fig. 2.71. Surface and radiographic anatomy extensor tendons. TS, probe transverse over dorsum of hand at metacarpal head.

Abdomen and pelvis

Anterior wall

Rectus sheath

- Aponeurosis of three muscles (external oblique, internal oblique, transversalis) to form linea alba in midline.

Proximal attachment

- Costal margin, xiphisternum.

Distal attachment

- Pubic symphysis and crest.

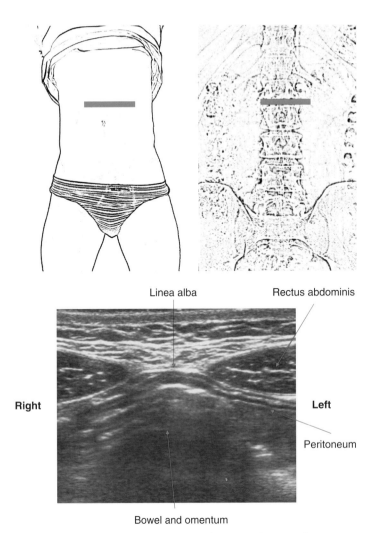

Linea alba   Rectus abdominis

Right   **Left**

Peritoneum

Bowel and omentum

Fig. 3.1. Surface and radiographic anatomy of the linea alba. TS, midline superior to umbilicus.

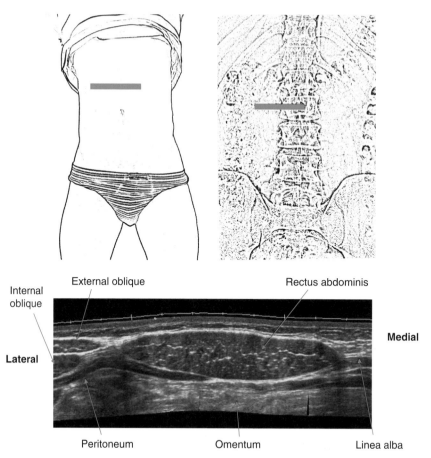

Fig. 3.2. Surface and radiographic anatomy of the rectus abdominis. TS, probe right of midline.

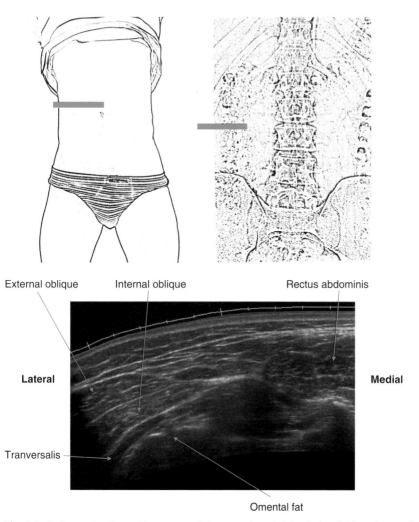

Fig. 3.3. Surface and radiographic anatomy of the antero-lateral abdominal wall. TS, probe over flank/anterior abdominal wall.

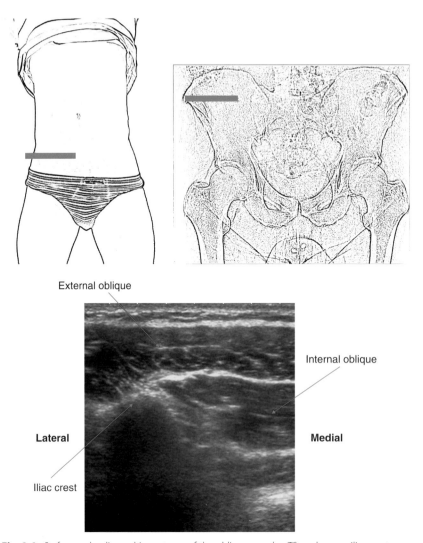

Fig. 3.4. Surface and radiographic anatomy of the oblique muscles. TS, probe over iliac crest.

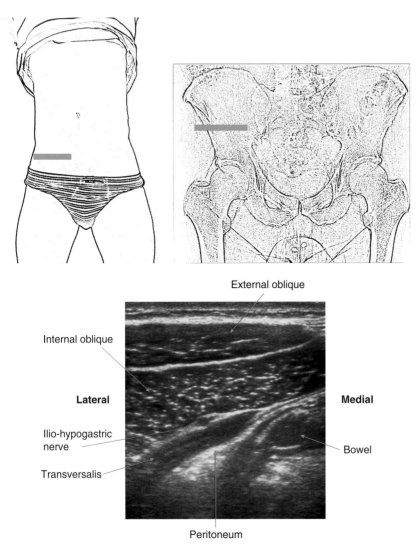

External oblique

Internal oblique

Lateral

Medial

Ilio-hypogastric
nerve

Bowel

Transversalis

Peritoneum

Fig. 3.5. Surface and radiographic anatomy of the ilio-hypogastric nerve. TS, oblique muscles.

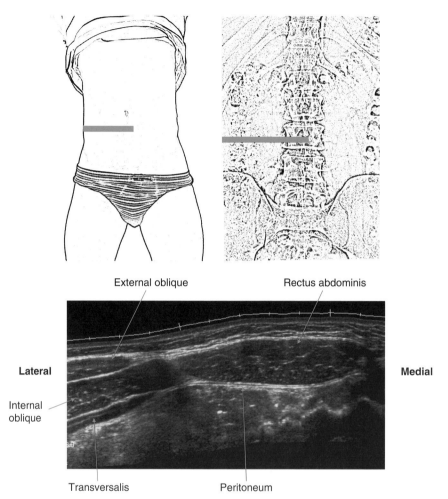

Fig. 3.6. Surface and radiographic anatomy of the rectus sheath. TS, panorama rectus sheath.

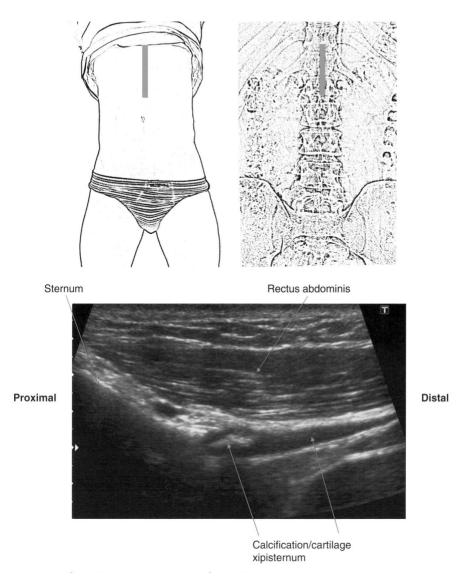

Sternum

Rectus abdominis

Proximal

Distal

Calcification/cartilage
xipisternum

Fig. 3.7. Surface and radiographic anatomy of the xiphisternum. LS, proximal rectus abdominis insertion and xiphisternum.

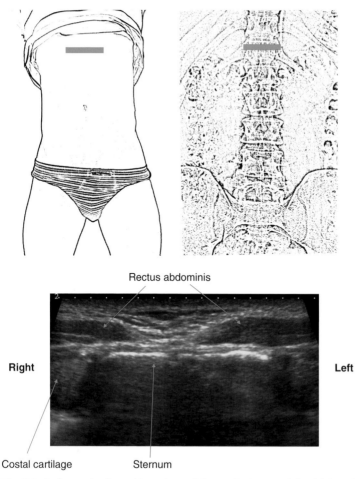

Rectus abdominis

Right

Left

Costal cartilage

Sternum

Fig. 3.8. Surface and radiographic anatomy of the proximal rectus abdominis insertion. TS, probe over xiphisternum. Proximal insertion is normally ill-defined and appearance of xiphisternum depends on the degree of calcification.

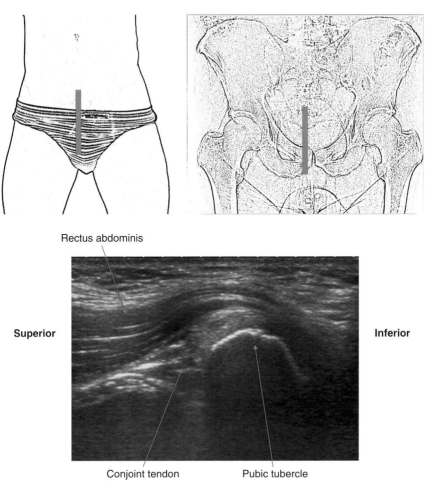

Rectus abdominis

Superior

Inferior

Conjoint tendon   Pubic tubercle

Fig. 3.9. Surface and radiographic anatomy of the distal rectus insertion. LS, probe over symphysis pubis.

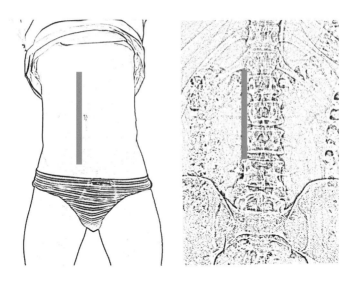

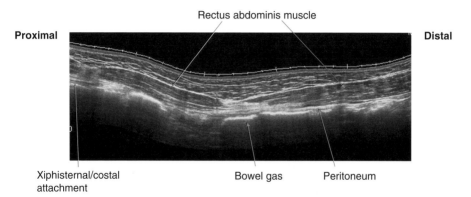

Proximal

Distal

Rectus abdominis muscle

Xiphisternal/costal
attachment

Bowel gas

Peritoneum

Fig. 3.10. Surface and radiographic anatomy of rectus abdominis. LS, panorama rectus abdominis.

Posterior wall

Thoracolumbar fascia – encloses muscles of posterior wall (erector spinae, latissimus dorsi, quadratus lumborum). Consists of three layers which fuse laterally with internal oblique and transversalis.

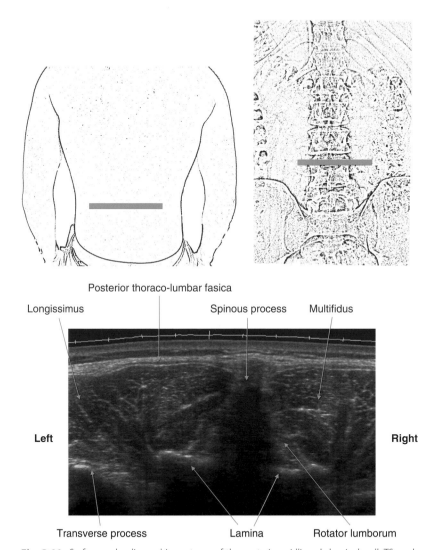

Fig. 3.11. Surface and radiographic anatomy of the posterior midline abdominal wall. TS, probe upper lumbar area midline.

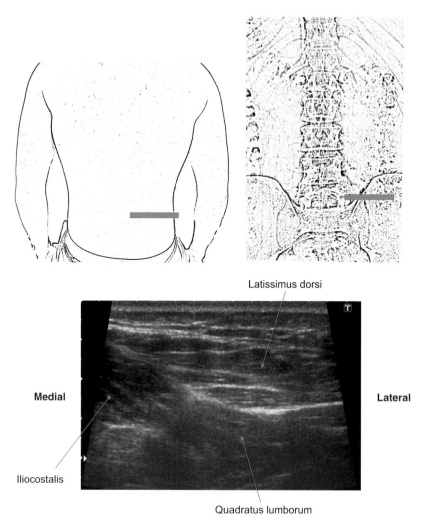

Latissimus dorsi

Medial   Lateral

Iliocostalis

Quadratus lumborum

Fig. 3.12. Surface and radiographic anatomy of the lumbar triangle. TS, probe right of midline, lumbar triangle.

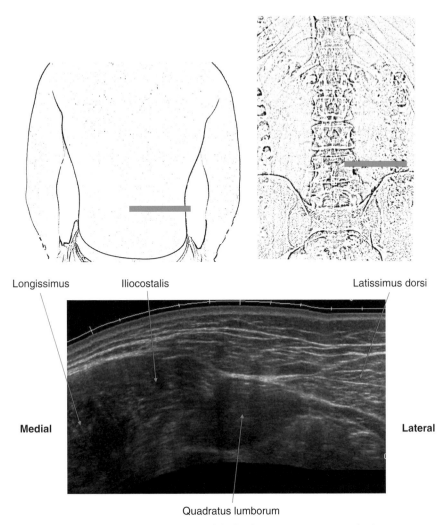

Fig. 3.13. Surface and radiographic anatomy of the lumbar region. TS, panorama lumbar region.

Groin

Inguinal ligament

- The lower free border of the external oblique aponeurosis between pubic tubercle and anterior superior iliac spine.

Inguinal canal

- Anterior wall: external oblique aponeurosis, reinforced by internal oblique.
- Posterior wall: transversalis fascia, reinforced by conjoint tendon medially.

Contents

Spermatic cord or round ligament, genito-femoral, ilio-inguinal and sympathetic nerves, testicular, cremasteric, and ductus deferens arteries.

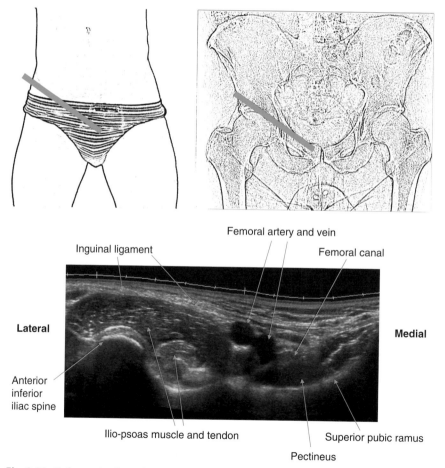

Fig. 3.14. Surface and radiographic anatomy of the inguinal ligament. TS, panorama along inguinal ligament.

Femoral triangle: boundaries

- Superior: inguinal ligament.
- Lateral: sartorius.
- Medial: adductor longus.
- Floor: adductor longus and pectineus.

Contents

- Femoral sheath, femoral nerve.
- Femoral sheath is a downward extension of the extraperitoneal fascia into the thigh.

Contents

- Lateral: femoral artery.
- Central: femoral vein.
- Medial: fat, lymphatics (femoral canal). This communicates superiorly via the femoral ring with abdominal extraperitoneal fascia.

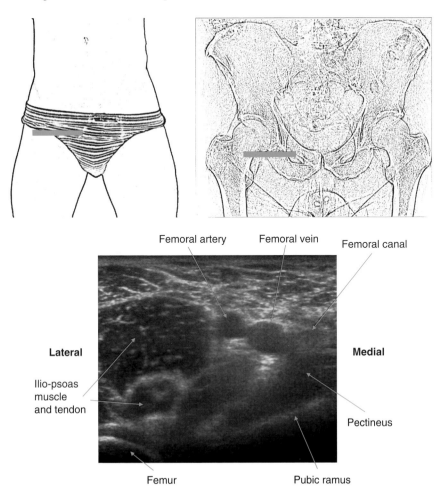

Fig. 3.15. Surface and radiographic anatomy of the femoral triangle. TS, femoral triangle. Leg abducted or adducted.

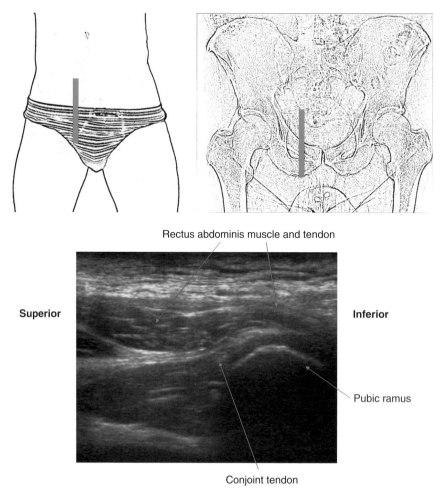

Rectus abdominis muscle and tendon

Superior

Inferior

Pubic ramus

Conjoint tendon

Fig. 3.16. Surface and radiographic anatomy of the rectus insertion/conjoint tendon. LS, probe over lateral aspect symphysis.

Symphysis pubis

United by fibrocartilaginous disc and interpubic ligaments.

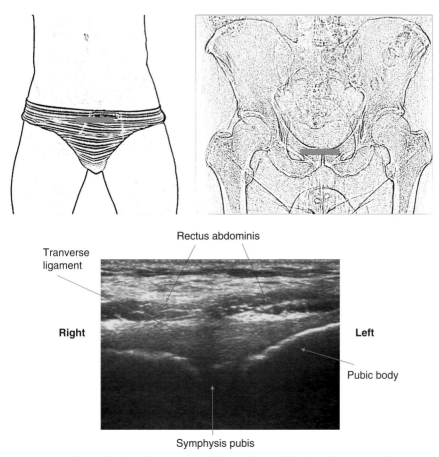

Fig. 3.17. Surface and radiographic anatomy of the symphysis pubis. TS, probe over symphysis.

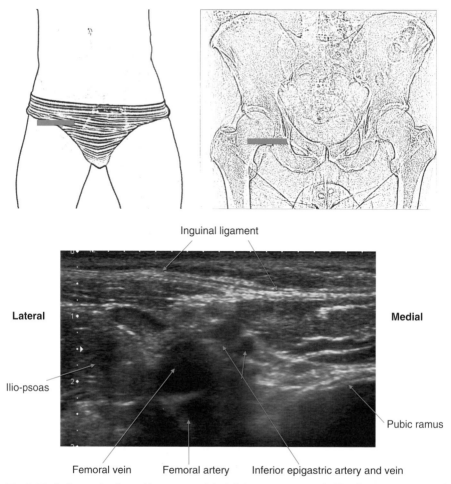

Lateral

Medial

Inguinal ligament

Ilio-psoas

Pubic ramus

Femoral vein   Femoral artery   Inferior epigastric artery and vein

Fig. 3.18. Surface and radiographic anatomy of the inferior epigastric vessels. TS, inferior epigastric vessels.

Conjoint tendon/superficial ring

The superficial ring is a deficiency in the transversalis fascia, at the midpoint of the inguinal ligament, lateral to the conjoint tendon and medial to the inferior epigastric vessels.

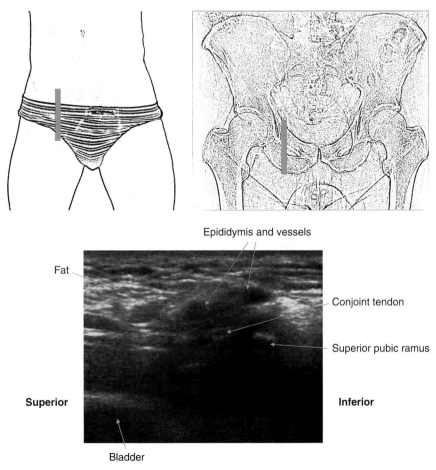

Fig. 3.19. Surface and radiographic anatomy of the conjoint tendon/superficial ring. LS, probe lateral to rectus tendon.

Deep ring: lateral to inferior epigastric vessels

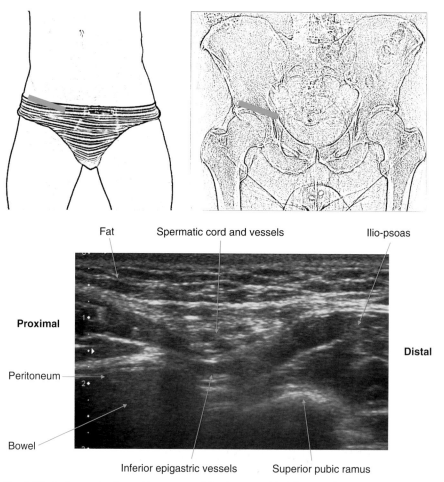

Fig. 3.20. Surface and radiographic anatomy of the deep ring. LS, oblique, probe superior to inguinal ligament angled parallel to ligament.

Femoral nerve

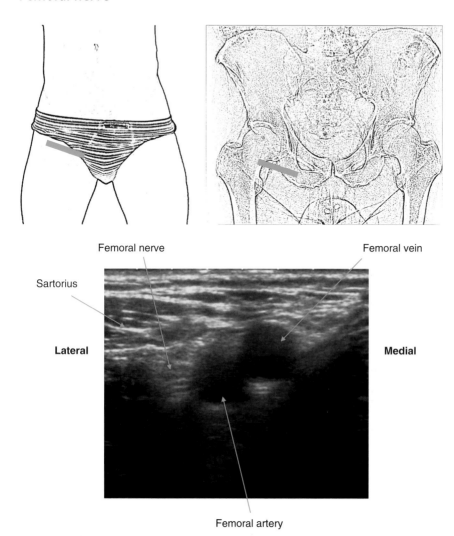

Fig. 3.21. Surface and radiographic anatomy of the femoral nerve. TS, over femoral vessels.

Lateral cutaneous nerve of the thigh

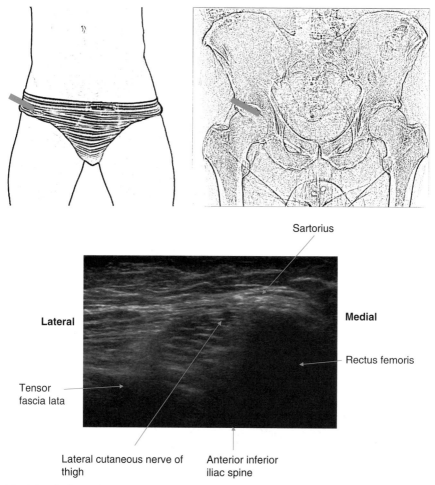

Sartorius

Lateral

Medial

Rectus femoris

Tensor
fascia lata

Lateral cutaneous nerve of
thigh

Anterior inferior
iliac spine

Fig. 3.22. Surface and radiographic anatomy of the lateral cutaneous nerve of the thigh. TS, probe over anterior inferior iliac spine/rectus femoris origin.

Ilio-hypogastric nerve

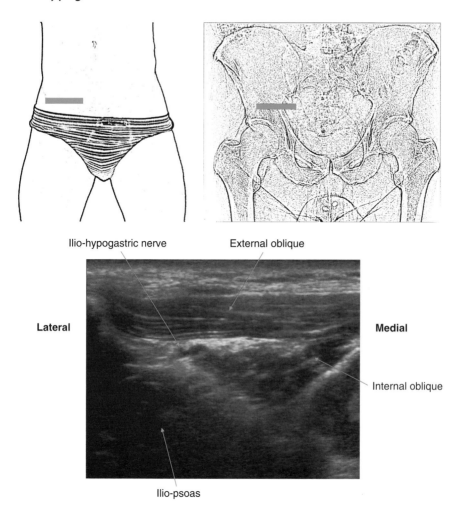

Ilio-hypogastric nerve   External oblique

Lateral   Medial

Internal oblique

Ilio-psoas

Fig. 3.23. Surface and radiographic anatomy of the ilio-hypogastric nerve. TS, probe over the oblique muscles.

Ilio-inguinal nerve

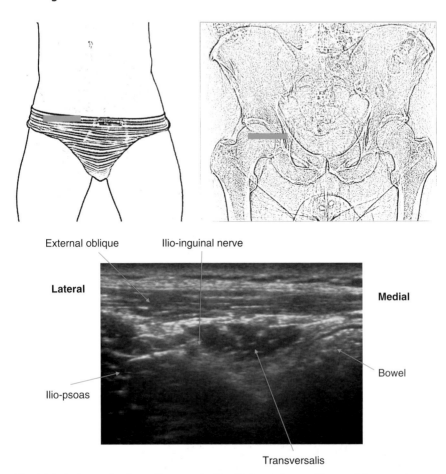

External oblique   Ilio-inguinal nerve

Lateral

Medial

Ilio-psoas

Bowel

Transversalis

Fig. 3.24. Surface and radiographic anatomy of the ilio-inguinal nerve. TS, over oblique muscles.

Pelvis and hip

Hip
Synovial ball and socket joint
Anterior

- Ilio-psoas and pectineus separate joint from femoral vessels and nerve.

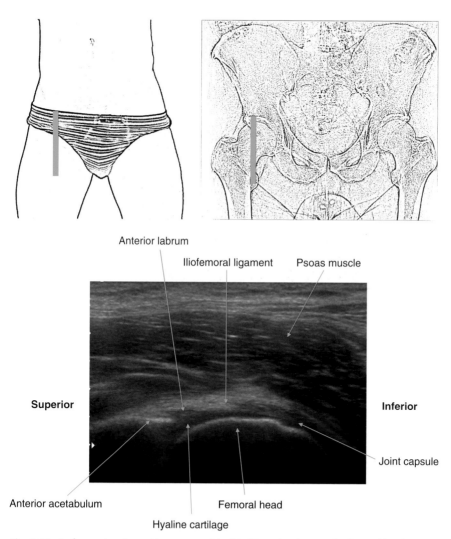

Fig. 3.25. Surface and radiographic anatomy of the hip. LS, supine, leg straight. Femoral head – LS.

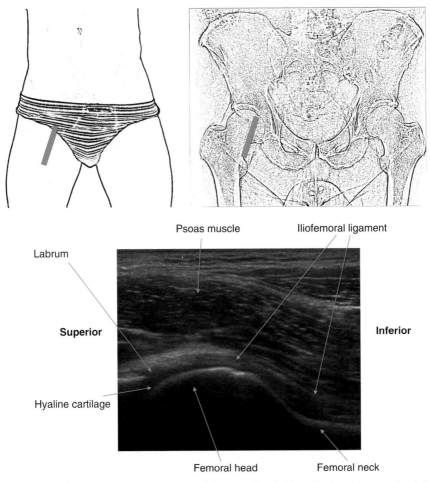

Fig. 3.26. Surface and radiographic anatomy of the femoral neck. LS, supine, leg straight, probe slightly distal to femoral head, angled to femoral neck.

Ilio-psoas

- Distal insertion: lesser trochanter.

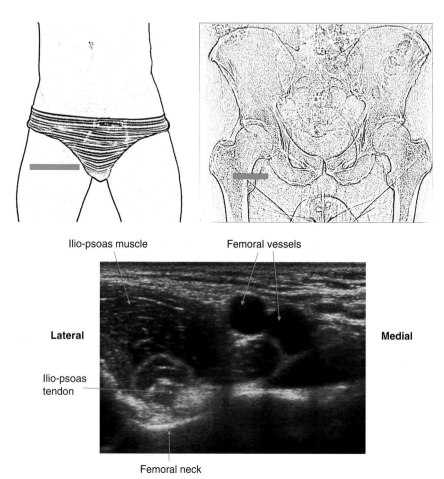

Fig. 3.27. Surface and radiographic anatomy of the ilio-psoas tendon. TS, probe proximal to the lesser trochanter.

- Distal psoas tendon.

  Difficulty due to anisotropy causing a hypoechoic appearance.

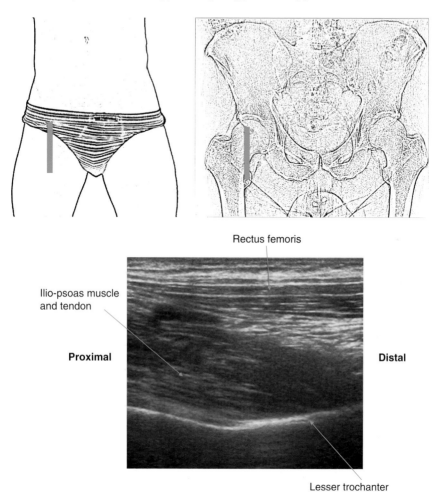

Fig. 3.28. Surface and radiographic anatomy of the distal psoas tendon. LS, probe over lesser trochanter.

Antero-lateral pelvis

- Sartorius: proximal attachment is at the anterior superior iliac spine, distal insertion is antero-medial tibia.

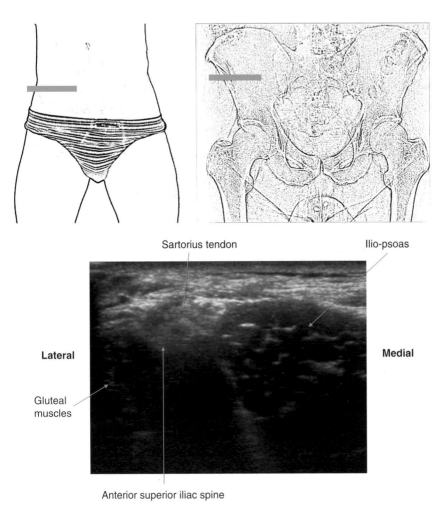

Fig. 3.29. Surface and radiographic anatomy of the proximal sartorius. TS, supine, leg straight probe over anterior superior iliac spine.

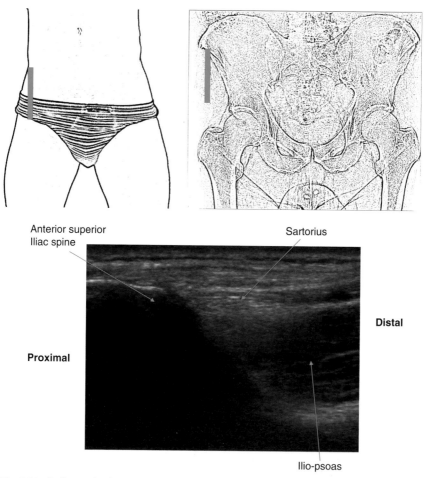

Fig. 3.30. Surface and radiographic anatomy of sartorius origin. LS, sartorius origin – probe over anterior superior iliac spine.

Rectus femoris

- Origin: anterior inferior iliac spine and ilium superolateral to the acetabulum.
- Insertion: upper border of patella.

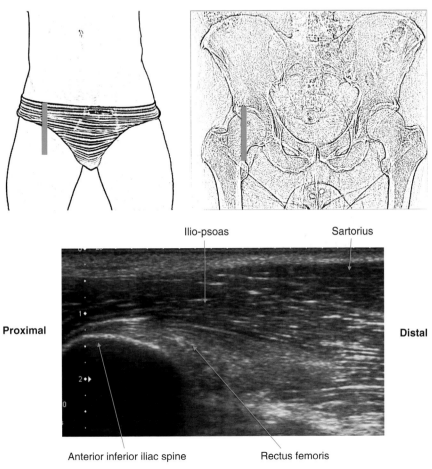

Ilio-psoas   Sartorius

Proximal   Distal

Anterior inferior iliac spine   Rectus femoris

Fig. 3.31. Surface and radiographic anatomy of the rectus femoris. LS, supine, proximal to hip joint over anterior inferior iliac spine.

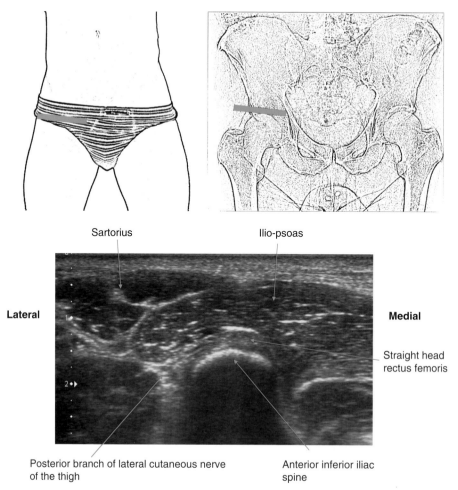

Sartorius   Ilio-psoas

Lateral   Medial

Straight head
rectus femoris

Posterior branch of lateral cutaneous nerve   Anterior inferior iliac
of the thigh   spine

Fig. 3.32. Surface and radiographic anatomy of the rectus femoris. TS, supine, proximal to hip joint over anterior inferior iliac spine.

Panorama anterior hip

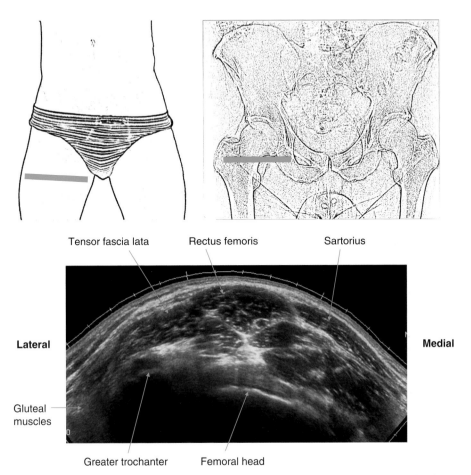

Fig. 3.33. Surface and radiographic anatomy of the anterior hip. TS, supine probe over femoral head.

Lateral hip
Greater trochanter
Fascia lata
- Origin: iliac crest.
- Insertion: ilio-tibial tract.

Gluteus maximus
- Origin: ilium, sacrum, coccyx.
- Insertion: ilio-tibial tract, gluteal tuberosity of femur.

Trochanteric bursa
- Deep to fascia lata and gluteus maximus.

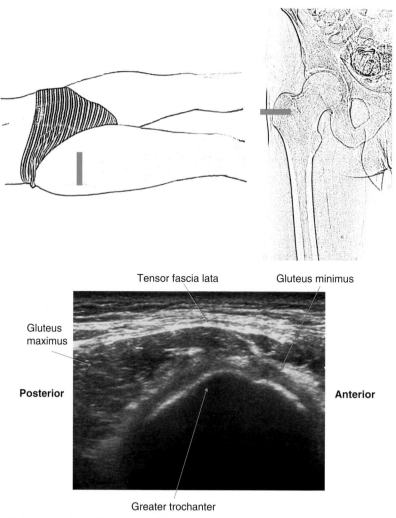

Fig. 3.34. Surface and radiographic anatomy of the greater trochanter. TS, supine, probe lateral overlying greater trochanter.

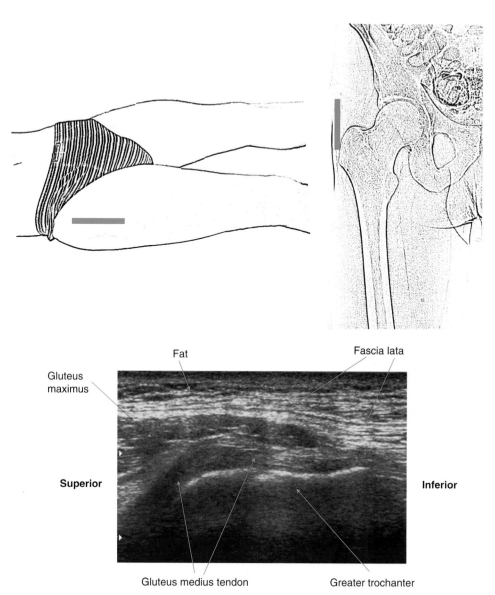

Fig. 3.35. Surface and radiographic anatomy of the abductor tendon insertion. LS, probe over greater trochanter.

Medial hip

Adductors

- Extend from adductor origin (pubis) into anteromedial thigh.

Pectineus

- Origin: pectineal line of the pubis to lesser trochanter/linea aspera.

Adductor longus

- Anterior pubis to linea aspera.

Adductor brevis

- Body and inferior ramus of pubis to linea aspera.

Adductor magnus

- Inferior pubic ramus and ischial tuberosity to linea aspera and adductor tubercle on medial femoral condyle.

Gracilis

- Pubic symphysis to antero-medial tibia.

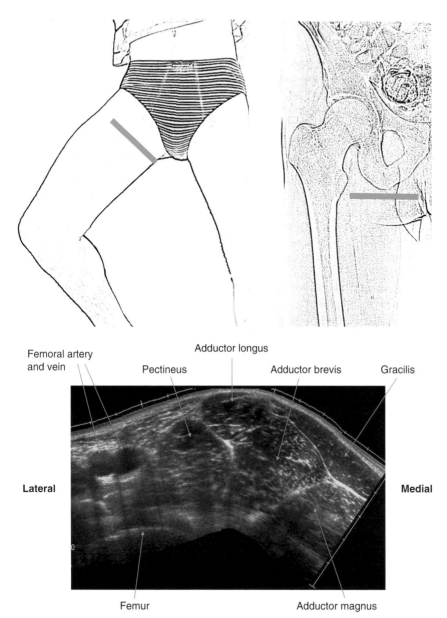

Fig. 3.36. Surface and radiographic anatomy of the adductors. TS, probe antero-medial thigh. The leg may be semi-flexed and abducted as an alternative position.

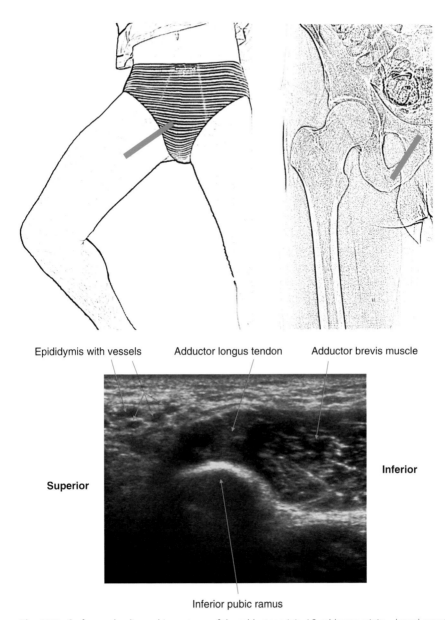

Epididymis with vessels   Adductor longus tendon   Adductor brevis muscle

Superior

Inferior

Inferior pubic ramus

Fig. 3.37. Surface and radiographic anatomy of the adductor origin. LS, adductor origin – lateral margin. LS, leg abducted.

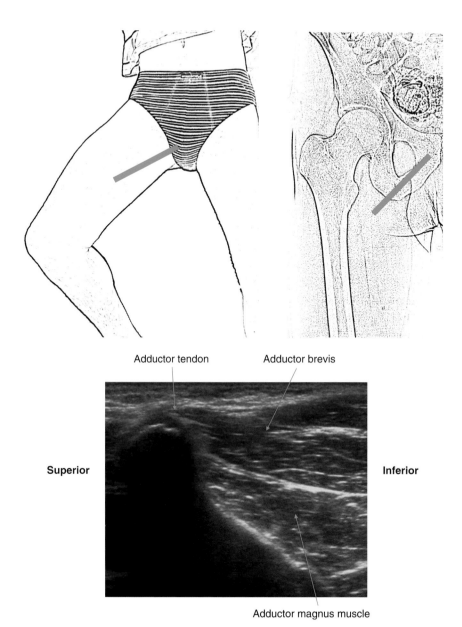

Adductor tendon   Adductor brevis

Superior   Inferior

Adductor magnus muscle

Fig. 3.38. Surface and radiographic anatomy of the adductor magnus. LS, adductor origin – probe medial margin, leg abducted.

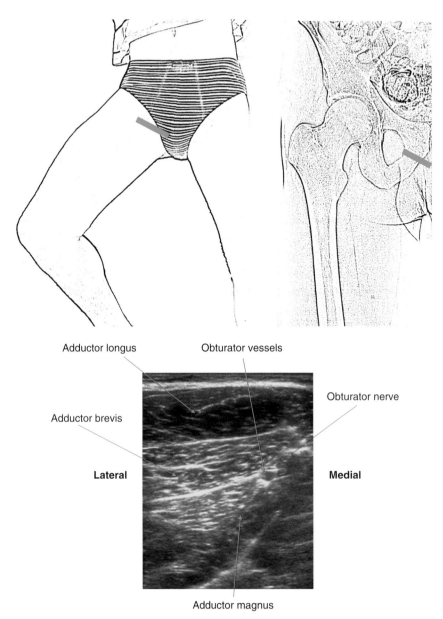

Fig. 3.39. Surface and radiographic anatomy of the adductors. TS, leg abducted.

Obturator nerve – proximal thigh

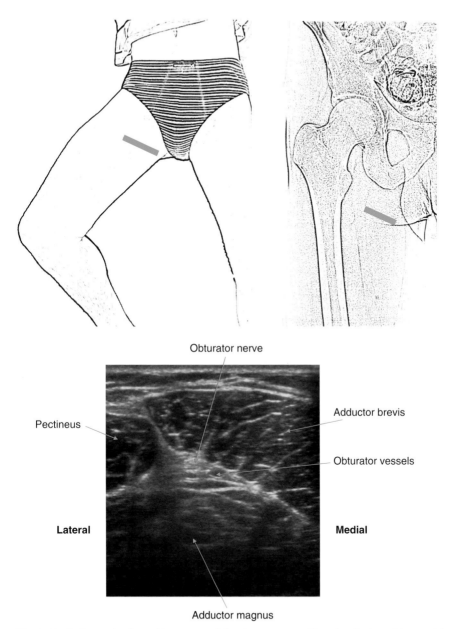

Obturator nerve

Pectineus

Adductor brevis

Obturator vessels

Lateral

Medial

Adductor magnus

Fig. 3.40. Surface and radiographic anatomy of the obturator nerve. TS, probe distal to adductor origins.

Posterior hip
Hamstring

- Origin.
- Semi-membranosus: ischial tuberosity.
- Biceps femoris and semi-tendinosus: common tendon from the ischial tuberosity (short head of biceps from linea aspera).

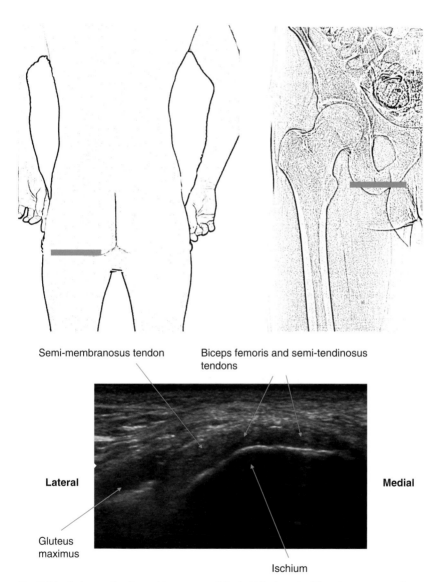

Fig. 3.41. Surface and radiographic anatomy of the ischial tuberosity. TS, patient prone, probe over ischial tuberosity.

Hamstring

- Origin LS.

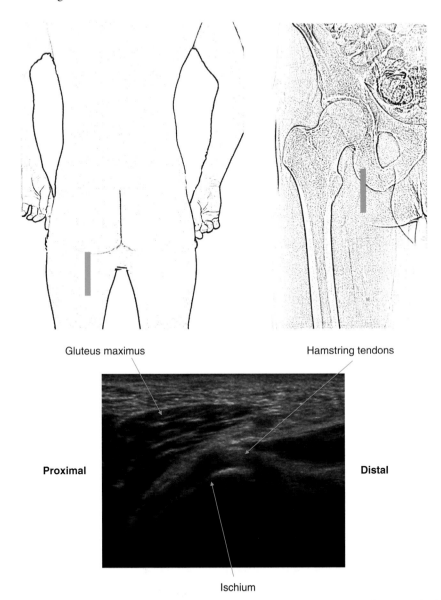

Fig. 3.42. Surface and radiographic anatomy of the hamstring origin. LS, prone, probe over mid ischial tuberosity.

Sciatic nerve lateral to ischium

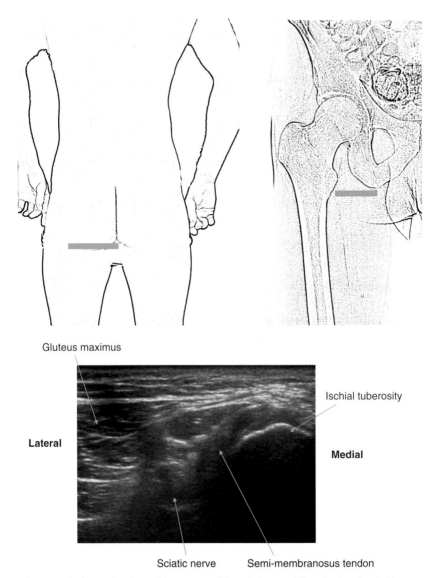

Fig. 3.43. Surface and radiographic anatomy of the sciatic nerve. TS, probe lateral to ischium.

Lower limb

Thigh

Anterior

Sartorius

- Origin: anterior superior iliac spine.
  – insertion, antero-medial tibia.

Quadriceps

- Rectus femoris: origin – anterior inferior iliac spine and ilium.
- Vastus lateralis: origin – greater trochanter and linea aspera.
- Vastus medialis: origin – linea aspera and lesser trochanter.
- Vastus intermedius: origin – anterior and lateral surface of femur.

The quadriceps muscles insert onto the upper pole of the patella.

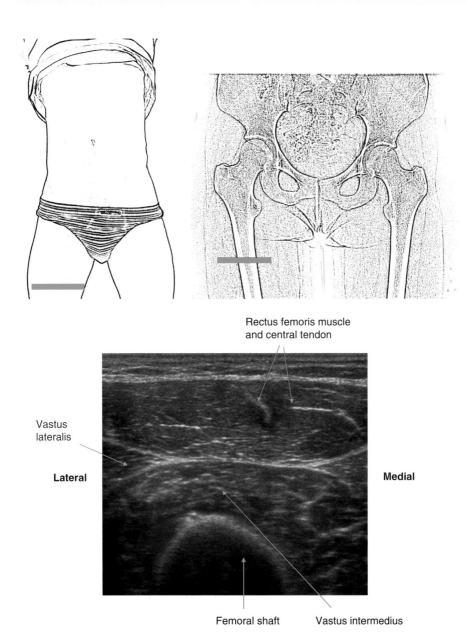

Fig. 4.1. Surface and radiographic anatomy of the rectus femoris. TS, supine, probe over anterior proximal thigh.

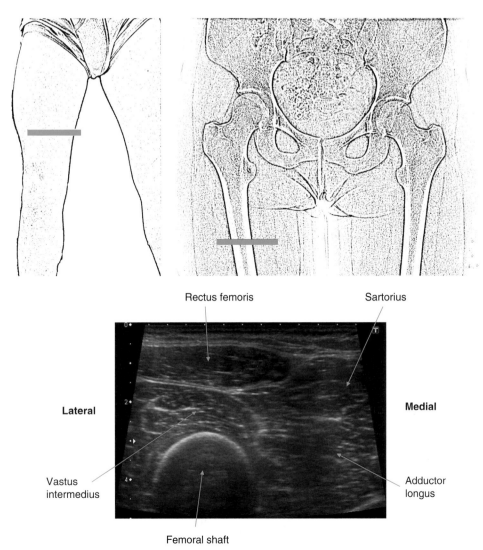

Rectus femoris   Sartorius

Lateral   Medial

Vastus   Adductor
intermedius   longus

Femoral shaft

Fig. 4.2. Surface and radiographic anatomy of the quadriceps. TS, supine anterior mid thigh.

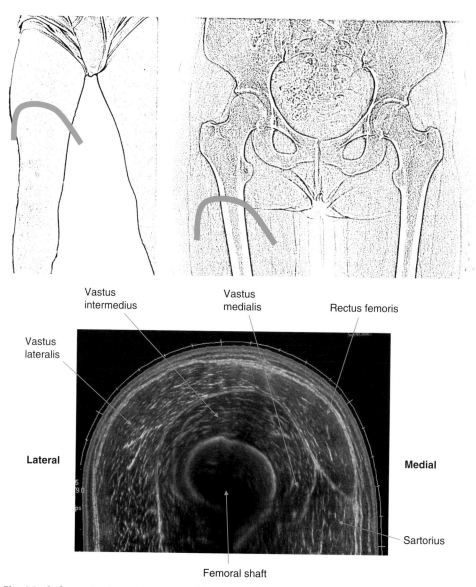

Fig. 4.3. Surface and radiographic anatomy of the anterior thigh. TS, panorama antero-lateral thigh.

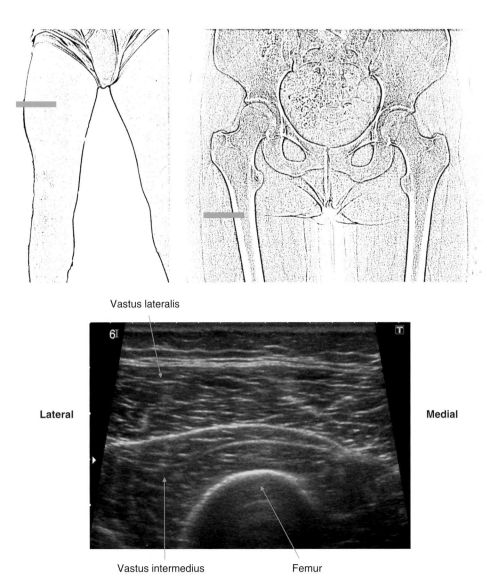

Fig. 4.4. Surface and radiographic anatomy of the antero-lateral thigh. TS, probe antero-lateral thigh.

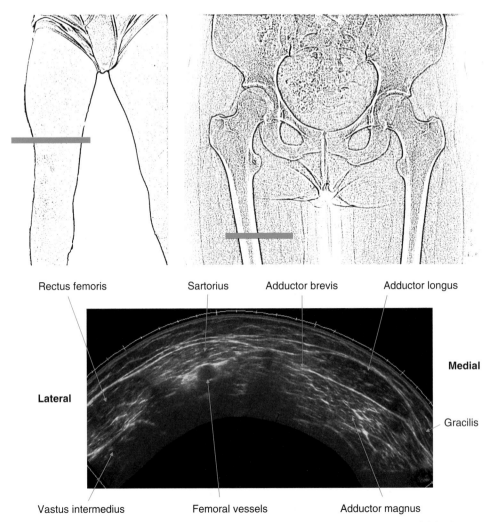

Fig. 4.5. Surface and radiographic anatomy of the antero-medial thigh. TS, panorama antero-medial thigh.

Thigh
Posterior
Hamstrings

- Semi-membranosus: insertion, postero-medial tibial condyle.
- Semi-tendinosus: insertion, medial tibia (pes anserinus).
- Biceps femoris: insertion, fibular apex.

The sciatic nerve is covered by gluteus maximus and hamstring muscles and lies on ischium, obturator internus, quadratus femoris, and adductor magnus.

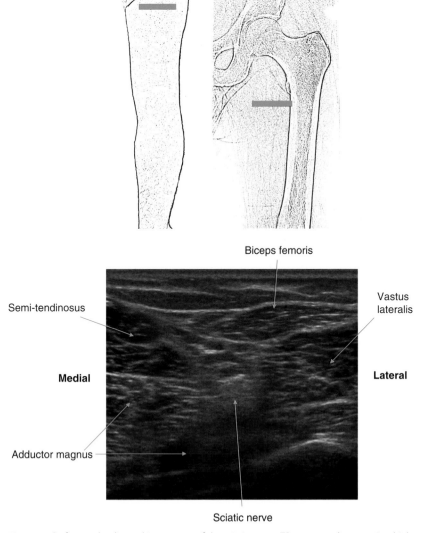

Fig. 4.6. Surface and radiographic anatomy of the sciatic nerve. TS, prone, probe posterior thigh.

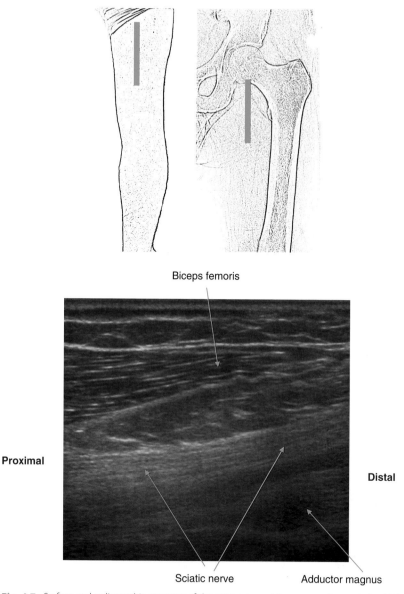

Fig. 4.7. Surface and radiographic anatomy of the sciatic nerve. LS, prone, probe posterior thigh.

Adductor canal

Femoral vessels pass through opening in adductor magnus just above adductor tubercle to the posterior knee.

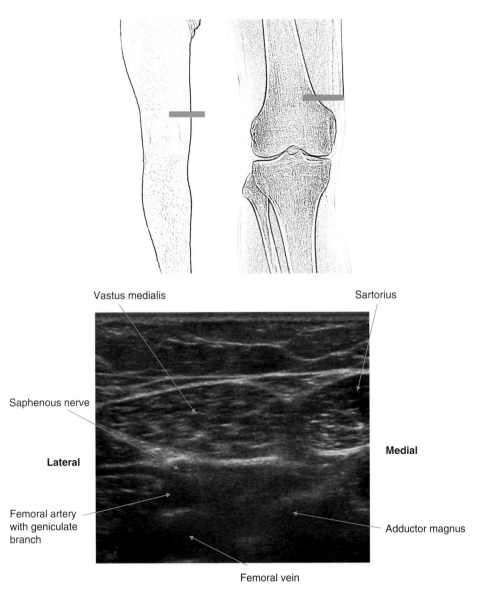

Fig. 4.8. Surface and radiographic anatomy of the adductor canal and saphenous nerve. TS, supine, probe antero-medial.

Knee

Modified hinge synovial joint.

Anterior knee

Quadriceps tendon – rectus femoris, vastus lateralis, medialis, intermedius.
Patella tendon – single musculotendinous expansion from lower patella to tibial tuberosity.

Bursae

- Superficial pre-patellar: superficial to lower patella and proximal patellar tendon.
- Deep infrapatellar: deep to patella tendon, separating it from tibia.

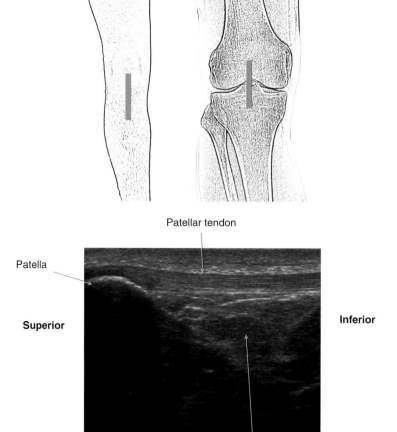

Fig. 4.9. Surface and radiographic anatomy of the patellar tendon. LS, probe at the level of the distal patella. Contract quads or flex knee to straighten tendon, avoiding anisotropy.

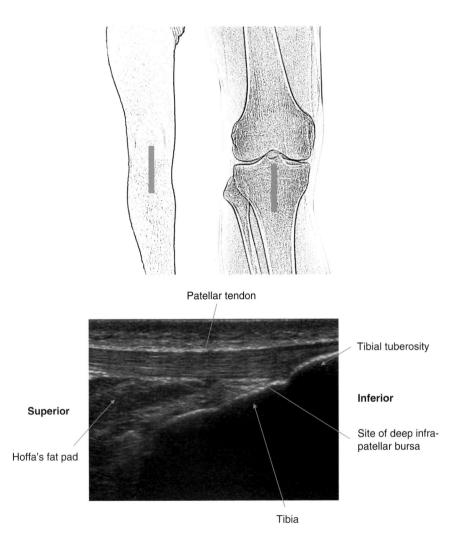

Fig. 4.10. Surface and radiographic anatomy of the distal patellar tendon. LS, probe distal patellar tendon insertion.

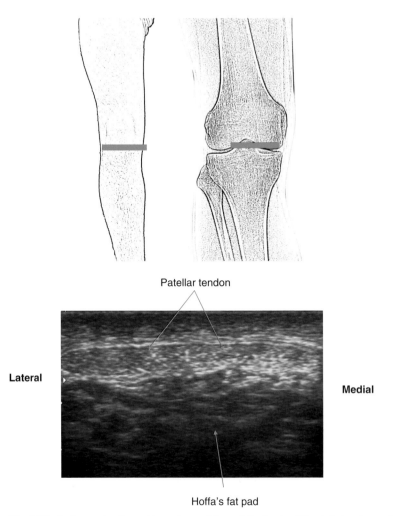

Fig. 4.11. Surface and radiographic anatomy of the patellar tendon. TS, patella tendon probe proximal to tibial tuberosity.

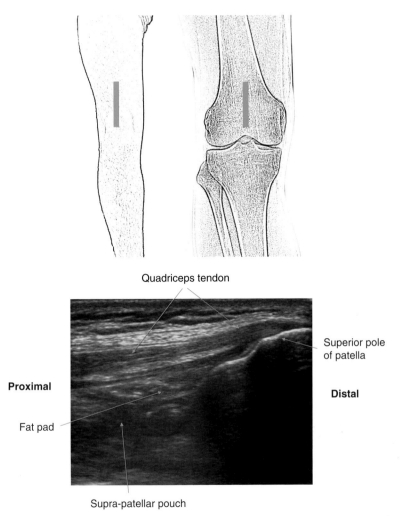

Quadriceps tendon

Superior pole
of patella

Proximal

Distal

Fat pad

Supra-patellar pouch

Fig. 4.12. Surface and radiographic anatomy of the quadriceps tendon. LS, probe proximal to the patella over the quadriceps tendon.

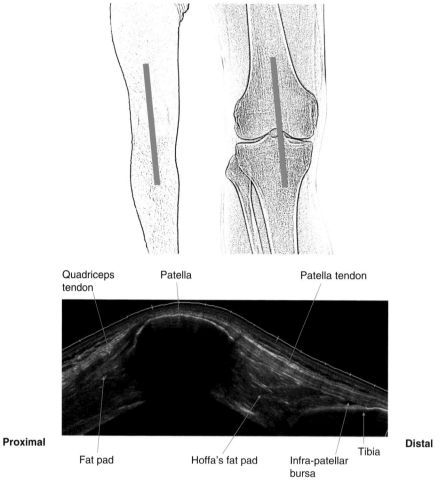

Fig. 4.13. Surface and radiographic anatomy of the extensor mechanism. LS, panorama extensor tendon.

Anterior cruciate ligament (ACL)

The ACL attaches on the antero-medial tibial intercondylar area and inserts on the medial surface of the lateral femoral condyle.

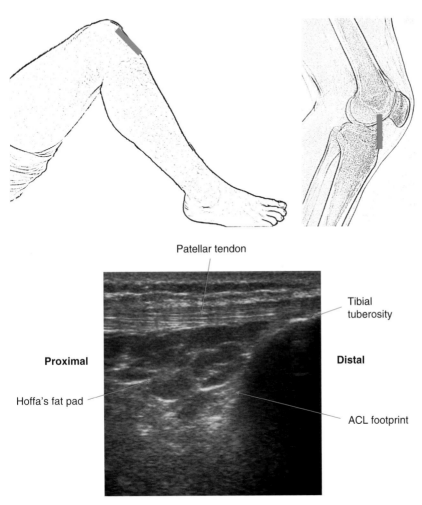

Fig. 4.14. Surface and radiographic anatomy of the anterior cruciate ligament. LS, probe over Hoffa's fat pad.

Trochlear groove

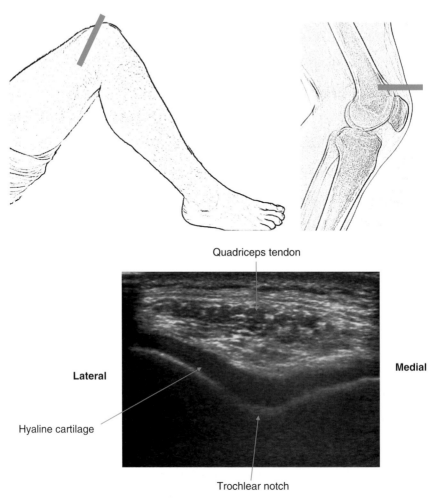

Quadriceps tendon

Lateral

Medial

Hyaline cartilage

Trochlear notch

Fig. 4.15. Surface and radiographic anatomy of the trochlear groove. TS, knee flexed, probe proximal to patella.

Antero-medial knee

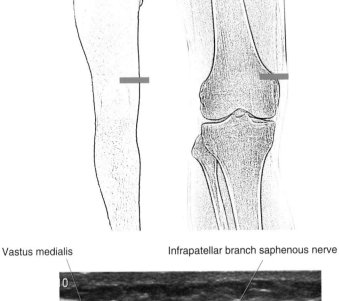

Vastus medialis

Infrapatellar branch saphenous nerve

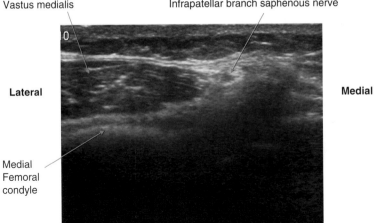

Lateral

Medial

Medial
Femoral
condyle

Fig. 4.16. Surface and radiographic anatomy of the infrapatellar branch of the saphenous nerve. TS, probe medial to patella.

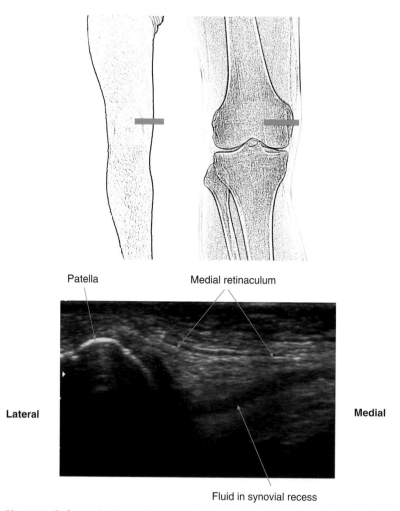

Fig. 4.17. Surface and radiographic anatomy of the medial patellar retinaculum. TS, probe medial to patella.

Pes anserinus

Insertion of sartorius, gracilis and semi-tendinosus. Semi-tendinosus inserts onto antero-medial tibia shaft, posterior to gracilis and sartorius. A bursa (bursa anserine) separates gracilis and semi-tendinosus from the tibia, with another bursa between them and sartorius.

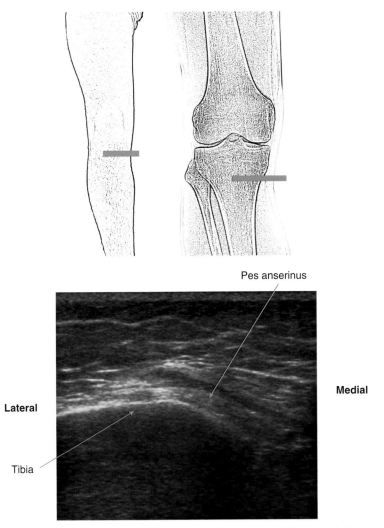

Fig. 4.18. Surface and radiographic anatomy of the pes anserinus. TS, leg extended, probe over antero-medial tibia. Semi-membranosus – inserts postero-medial tibial condyle.

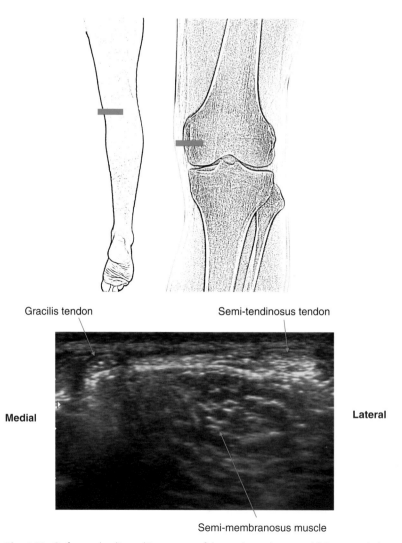

Fig. 4.19. Surface and radiographic anatomy of the semi-membranosus. LS, leg extended, prone, probe postero-medial knee.

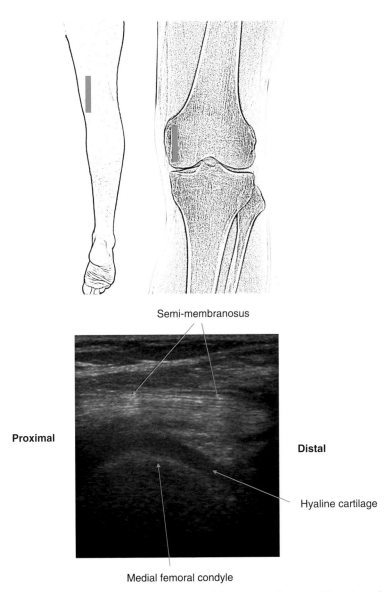

Semi-membranosus

Proximal

Distal

Hyaline cartilage

Medial femoral condyle

Fig. 4.20. Surface and radiographic anatomy of the semi-membranosus. LS, semi-membranosus tendon: postero-medial knee.

Medial knee

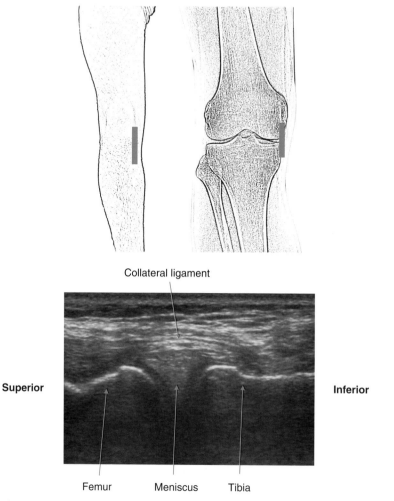

Fig. 4.21. Surface and radiographic anatomy of the medial meniscus. LS, leg straight, probe along medial joint line. Valgus strain may be applied to assess stability.

Medial collateral ligament

Approximately 10 cm in length, arises from the medial femoral epicondyle and extends to the proximal medial tibial shaft. Deeper layer is attached to the medial tibial condyle and blends with the medial meniscus.

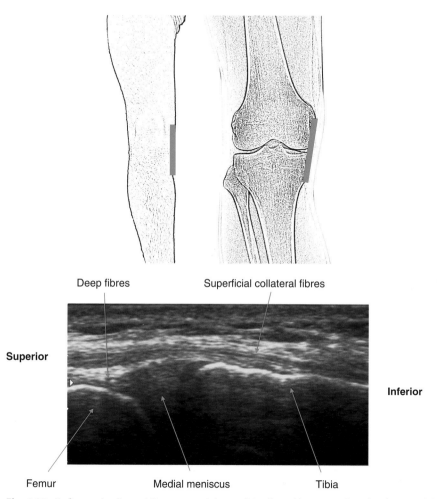

Deep fibres **Superficial collateral fibres**

Superior

Inferior

Femur Medial meniscus Tibia

Fig. 4.22. Surface and radiographic anatomy of the medial collateral ligament. LS, probe along medial joint line.

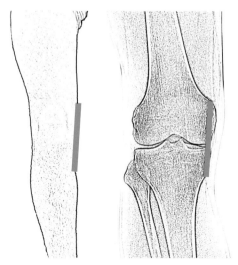

Proximal

Medial collateral ligament

Distal

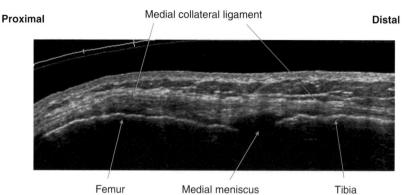

Femur   Medial meniscus   Tibia

Fig. 4.23. LS, panorama medial knee.

Lateral knee
Lateral collateral ligament
Arises from the lateral femoral epicondyle and extends to the apex of the fibula.

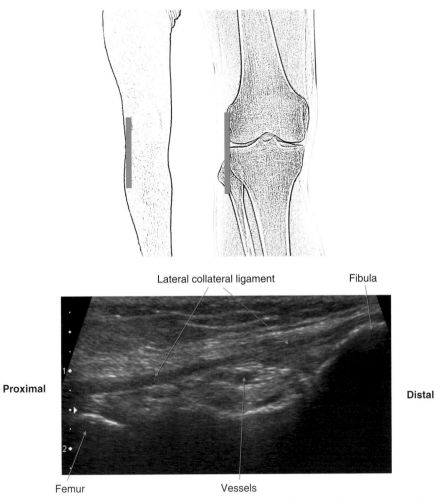

Fig. 4.24. Surface and radiographic anatomy of the lateral collateral ligament. LS, leg extended, probe over lateral joint line. Popliteus tendon deep to the lateral collateral ligament.

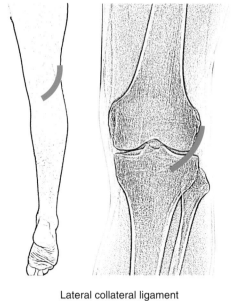

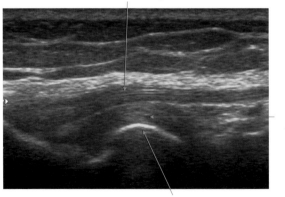

Lateral collateral ligament

Distal

Proximal

Popliteus
tendon

Lateral femoral condyle

Fig. 4.25. Surface and radiographic anatomy of the popliteus tendon. LS probe longitudinal to popliteus tendon.

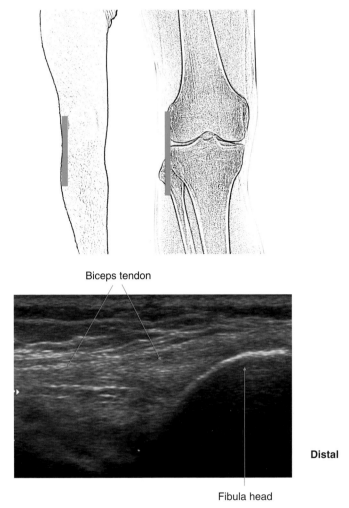

Biceps tendon

Proximal

Distal

Fibula head

Fig. 4.26. Surface and radiographic anatomy of the biceps insertion. LS, leg extended probe over fibular head.

Ilio-tibial tract

Broad thickening of the fascia lata arising from the outer lip of iliac crest and inserting on the antero-lateral aspect of tibia at Gerdy's tubercle. The gluteus maximus and tensor fasciae lata muscles attach to it.

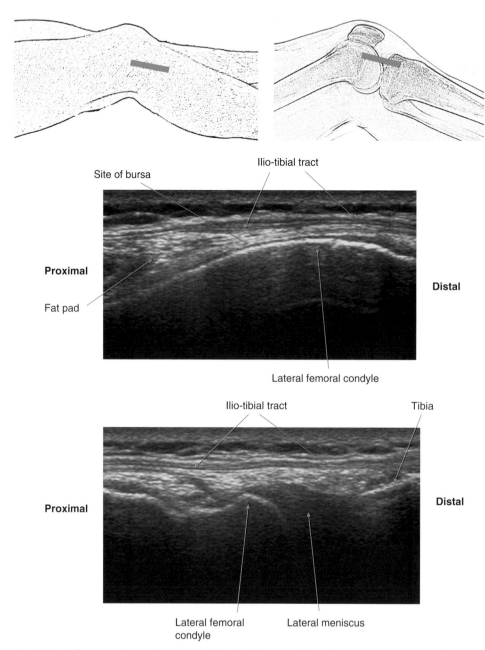

Fig. 4.27. Surface and radiographic anatomy of the ilio-tibial tract. LS, knee flexed, probe antero-lateral aspect. Leg flexed. Leg extended.

Common peroneal nerve

This is a terminal branch of the sciatic nerve formed just proximal to the popliteal fossa. It lies on the lateral head of gastrocnemius and then on the neck of the fibula and is deep to biceps femoris. It pierces peroneus longus to divide into superficial and deep branches.

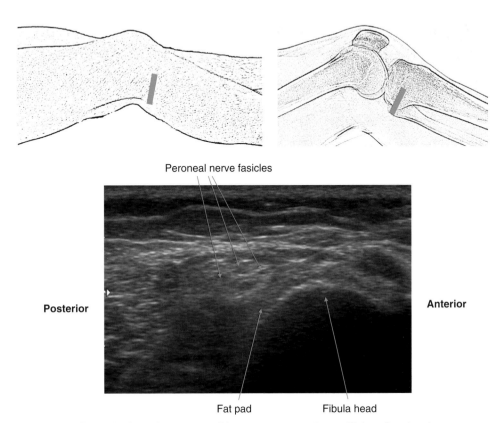

Fig. 4.28. Surface and radiographic anatomy of the common peroneal nerve. TS, knee flexed, probe over fibular neck.

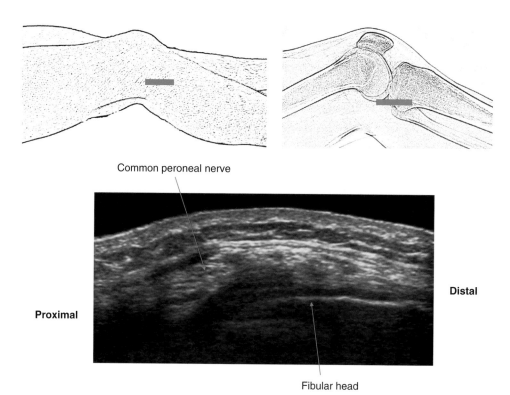

Fig. 4.29. Surface and radiographic anatomy of the peroneal nerve. LS, peroneal nerve.

Posterior knee
Popliteal fossa
Contents
Popliteal artery and vein and branches, tibial and common peroneal nerves, lymph nodes and fat.

Boundaries
- Lateral: biceps.
- Medial: semi-tendinosus, semi-membranosus.
- Inferior: medial and lateral heads of gastrocnemius.

Posterior cruciate ligament
Lateral surface of medial femoral condyle to posterior intercondylar area of tibia.

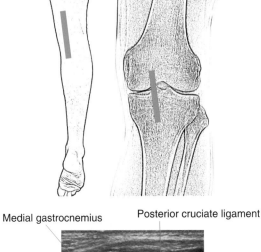

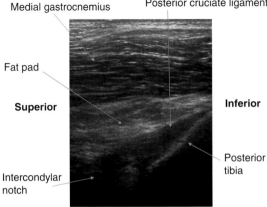

Fig. 4.30. Surface and radiographic anatomy of the posterior cruciate ligament. LS, posterior knee, medial popliteal fossa.

Lateral popliteal fossa

Biceps femoris attaches to apex of fibula.

Popliteus tendon arises from the lateral aspect of the lateral femoral condyle, and is attached to the lateral meniscus. The muscle attaches to the posterior tibia proximal to the soleal line. The popliteus bursa lies between the muscle and tibia.

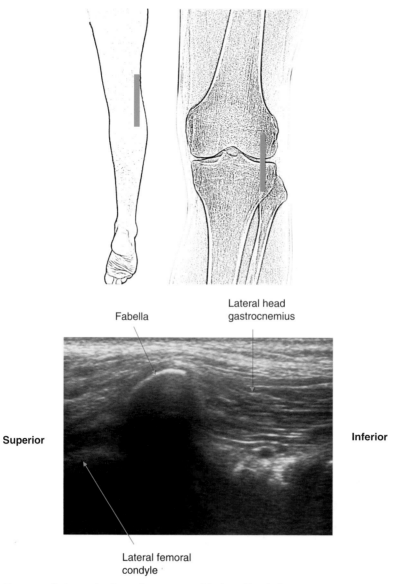

Fabella

Lateral head gastrocnemius

Superior

Inferior

Lateral femoral condyle

Fig. 4.31. Surface and radiographic anatomy of the lateral head of gastrocnemius. LS, probe over lateral popliteal fossa.

Popliteal fossa 'cyst space'

Cyst neck lies between medial head of gastrocnemius and semi-membranosus tendon.

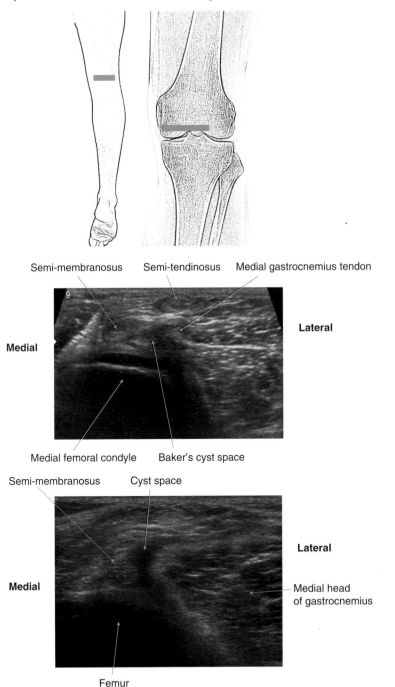

Fig. 4.32. Surface and radiographic anatomy of the 'cyst space'. TS, probe over medial head of gastrocnemius.

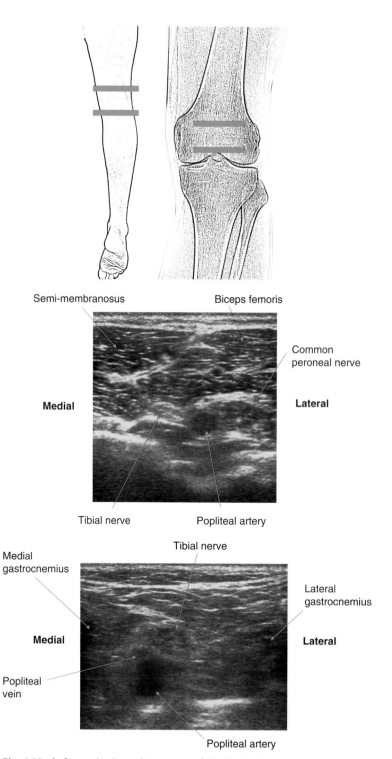

Fig. 4.33. Surface and radiographic anatomy of the tibial and common peroneal nerves. TS popliteal fossa.

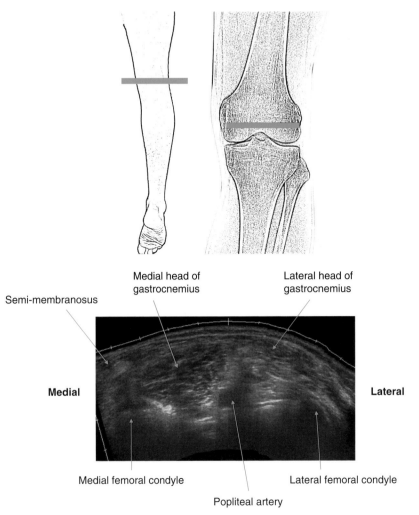

Fig. 4.34. Panorama of the popliteal fossa.

Calf

Anterior, lateral and posterior compartments divided by tibia and fibula, interosseous membrane, and anterior and posterior intermuscular septa. The anterior septum passes to the anterior border of the fibula and separates the anterior (dorsiflexor) from the lateral (evertor) compartment.

Tibialis anterior

- Origin: proximal two-thirds of tibia.
- Insertion: medial cuneiform and first metatarsal.

Extensor hallucis longus

- Origin: anterior proximal fibula.
- Insertion: distal phalanx great toe.

Extensor digitorum longus

- Origin: anterior proximal fibula, lateral condyle tibia and interosseous membrane.
- Insertion: dorsum of middle and terminal phalanges.

Peroneus tertius

- Origin: lower anterior fibula.
- Insertion: fifth metatarsal.

Antero-lateral compartment

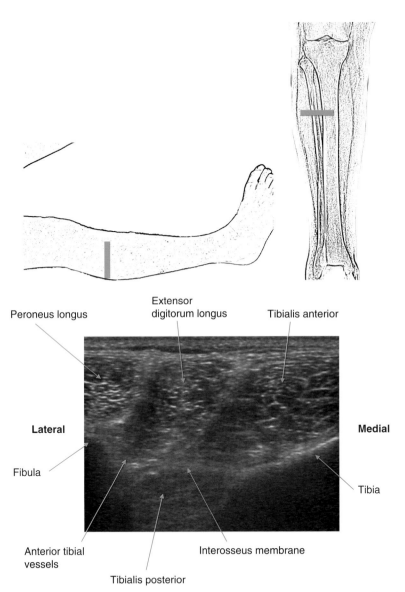

Peroneus longus

Extensor
digitorum longus

Tibialis anterior

Lateral

Fibula

Medial

Tibia

Anterior tibial
vessels

Interosseus membrane

Tibialis posterior

Fig. 4.35. Surface and radiographic anatomy of the extensor compartment. TS, probe lateral to tibia.

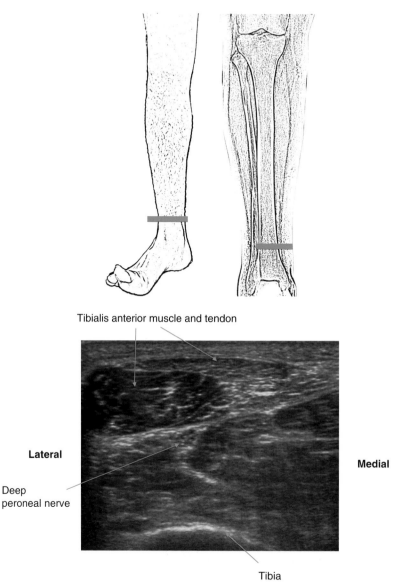

Tibialis anterior muscle and tendon

Lateral

Medial

Deep
peroneal nerve

Tibia

Fig. 4.36. Surface and radiographic anatomy of the tibialis anterior and deep peroneal nerve. TS, distal anterior calf.

Lateral compartment

Peroneus longus

- Origin: proximal lateral fibula.
- Insertion: first metatarsal and medial cuneiform.

Peroneus brevis

- Origin: lower lateral fibula.
- Insertion: fifth metatarsal.

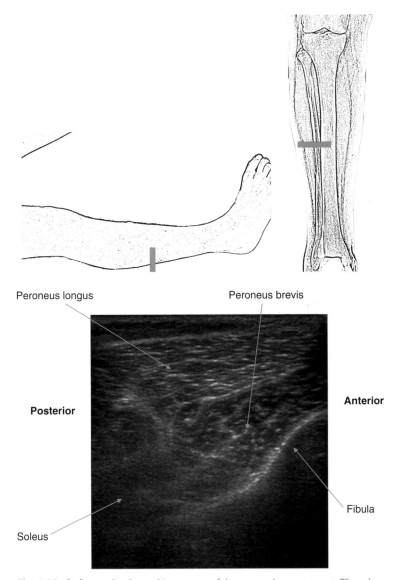

Fig. 4.37. Surface and radiographic anatomy of the peroneal compartment. TS, probe over lateral mid calf.

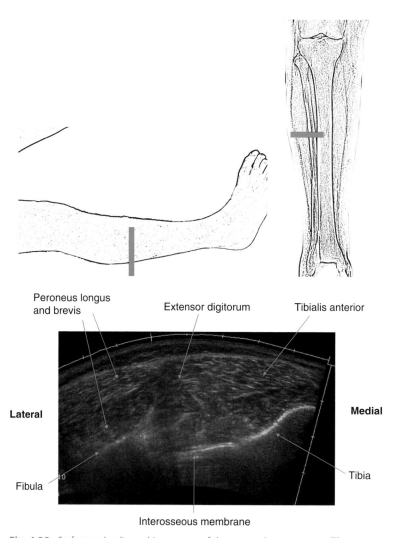

Peroneus longus and brevis

Extensor digitorum

Tibialis anterior

Lateral

Medial

Fibula

Tibia

Interosseous membrane

Fig. 4.38. Surface and radiographic anatomy of the peroneal compartment. TS, panorama antero-lateral compartment.

Posterior compartment
Superficial muscles
- Gastrocnemius

    Origin – medial and lateral femoral condyles.
    Insertion – soleus and tendo-achilles.

- Soleus

    Origin – soleal line tibia and posterior fibula.
    Insertion – tendo-achilles.

- Plantaris

    Origin – lateral supracondylar line.
    Insertion – tendo-achilles.

Deep muscles
- Popliteus

    Origin – posterior tibia proximal to soleal line.
    Insertion – lateral femoral epicondyle.

- Flexor digitorum longus

    Origin – medial posterior tibia.
    Insertion – terminal phalanges lateral four toes.

- Tibialis posterior

    Origin – posterior interosseus membrane, tibia and fibula.
    Insertion – navicular.

- Flexor hallicus longus

    Origin – posterior distal fibula.
    Insertion – distal phalanx great toe.

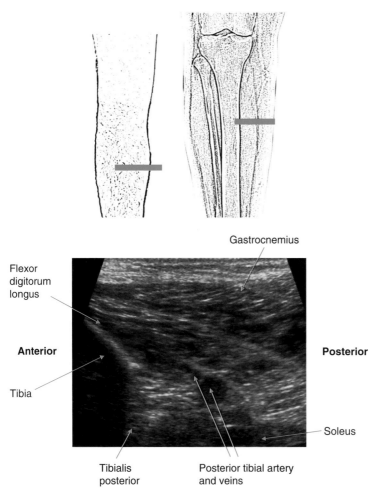

Fig. 4.39. Surface and radiographic anatomy of the medial compartment. TS, probe medial to tibia.

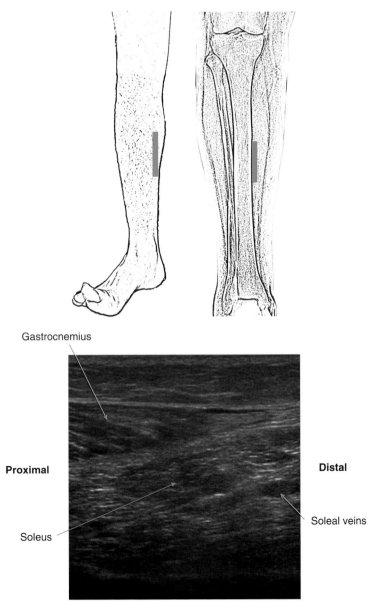

Fig. 4.40. Surface and radiographic anatomy of the medial gastrocnemius. LS, mid posterior calf.

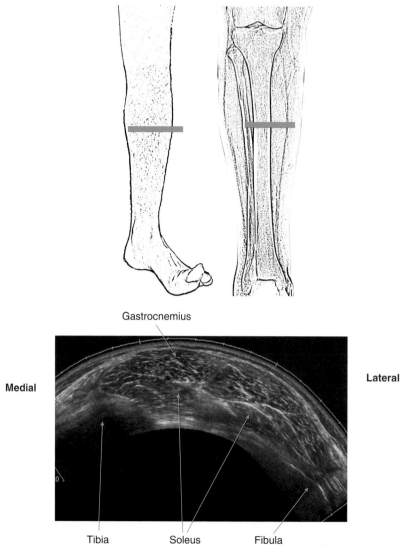

Fig. 4.41. Surface and radiographic anatomy of the posterior calf. TS, panorama proximal posterior calf.

Ankle: posterior

Tendo-achilles; formed by gastrocnemius and soleus to attach distally to the posterior superior calcaneum. There is no synovial sheath, but it has a hyperechoic paratenon. Deep to distal tendon is Kager's fat pad and pre-achilles bursa. Retro-achilles bursa lies posterior to the tendon attachment.

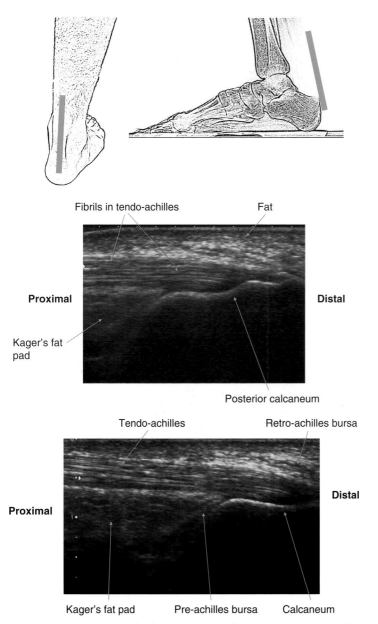

Fig. 4.42. LS, patient prone, distal insertion. Stand-off medium is sometimes useful. Dynamic examination should be performed by passively and actively dorsi- and plantar-flexing the foot. Dorsi-flexion straightens the tendon to avoid anisotropy.

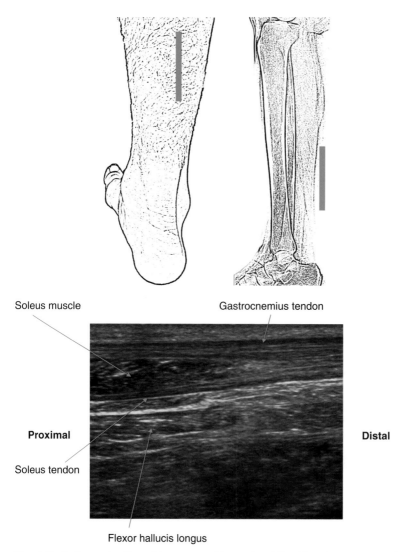

Soleus muscle   Gastrocnemius tendon

Proximal   **Distal**

Soleus tendon

Flexor hallucis longus

Fig. 4.43. Surface and radiographic anatomy of the tendo-achilles. LS, probe over proximal tendon.

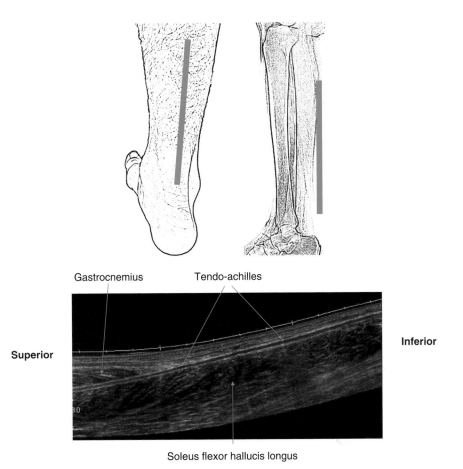

Gastrocnemius   Tendo-achilles

Superior

Inferior

Soleus flexor hallucis longus

Fig. 4.44. Surface and radiographic anatomy of the gastro soleus aponeurosis tendo-achilles. LS, patient prone.

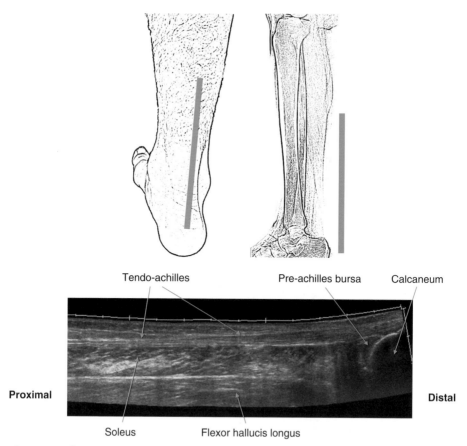

Fig. 4.45. Surface and radiographic anatomy of the proximal tendo-achilles. LS, panorama of distal tendo-achilles.

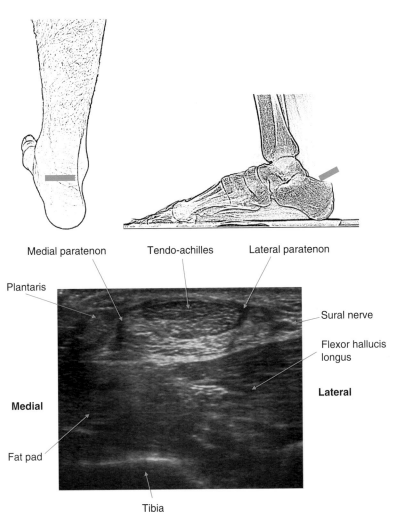

Medial paratenon   Tendo-achilles   Lateral paratenon

Plantaris

Sural nerve

Flexor hallucis
longus

Lateral

Medial

Fat pad

Tibia

Fig. 4.46. Surface and radiographic anatomy of the distal tendo-achilles. LS, probe over of distal tendo-achilles.

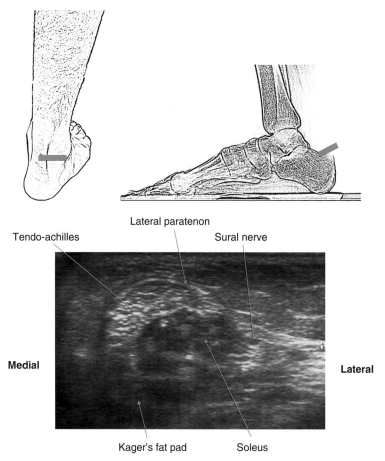

Medial

Lateral

Tendo-achilles

Lateral paratenon

Sural nerve

Kager's fat pad

Soleus

Fig. 4.47. Surface and radiographic anatomy of the lateral paratenon. TS, prone with probe over lateral tendo-achilles. Angle medially and laterally for paratenon. Due to edge effect, the medial and lateral paratenon is difficult to visualize unless the probe is angled to assess them individually. A stand-off pad is often helpful for assessment of the tendo-achilles. Surface and radiographic anatomy of the lateral paratenon. TS, probe angled over lateral tendon.

Ankle: lateral

Ligaments –antero-lateral ligament complex composed of three separate parts:

- calcaneo-fibular,
- posterior talo-fibular and
- anterior talo-fibular ligaments.

Posterior talo-fibular is not successfully imaged on ultrasound.

Calcaneo-fibular ligament

Passes posteriorly from the tip of the lateral malleolus to the lateral border of the calcaneum.

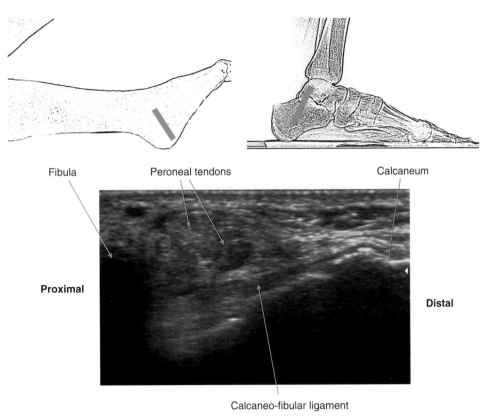

Fig. 4.48. Surface and radiographic anatomy of the calcaneo-fibular ligament. LS, foot may be internally rotated, probe posterior and inferior to lateral malleolus. Foot eversion and inversion for dynamic examination.

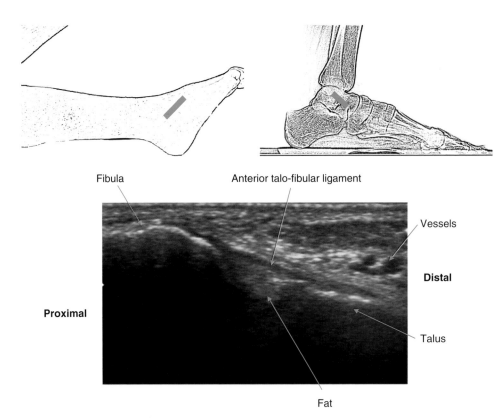

Fig. 4.49. Surface and radiographic anatomy of the anterior talo-fibular ligament. LS, probe anterior and inferior to lateral malleolus. Anterior talo-fibular ligament passes horizontally from lateral malleolus to neck of talus. Foot eversion and inversion for dynamic examination.

Tendons

Peroneus longus and brevis. Brevis is anterior to longus and both should be posterior to the lateral malleolus.

- Peroneus longus

    Origin – proximal lateral fibula.
    Insertion – first metatarsal and medial cuneiform.

- Peroneus brevis

    Origin – distal lateral fibula.
    Insertion – fifth metatarsal.

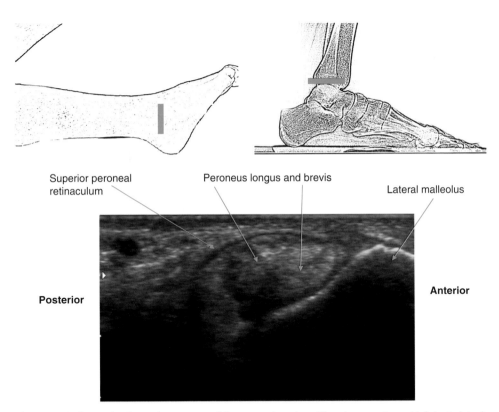

Fig. 4.50. Surface and radiographic anatomy of the peroneal tendons. TS, probe posterior and inferior to lateral malleolus. Plantar flexing the foot can 'straighten' the tendons. Dynamic examination using foot eversion and dorsiflexion.

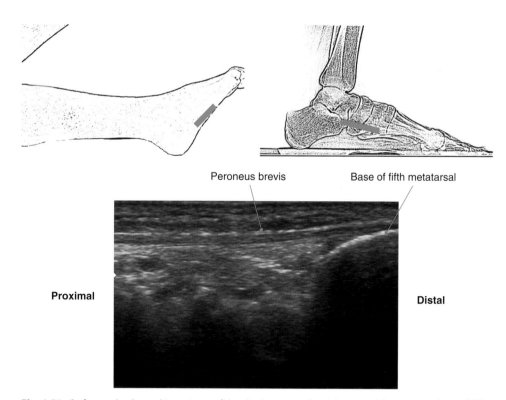

Peroneus brevis   Base of fifth metatarsal

Proximal   Distal

Fig. 4.51. Surface and radiographic anatomy of the distal peroneus brevis insertion. LS, probe over base of fifth metatarsal.

Ankle: medial
ligaments: deltoid

Deltoid ligament: triangular shaped with deep and superficial layers. The superficial part lies between tibia and navicular, spring ligament and calcaneum. The deep layer extends from medial malleolus to neck of talus.

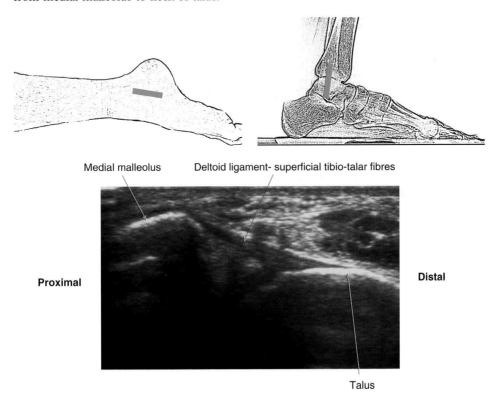

Medial malleolus   Deltoid ligament- superficial tibio-talar fibres

Proximal

Distal

Talus

Fig. 4.52. Surface and radiographic anatomy of the superficial fibres deltoid ligament. LS, probe inferior to medial malleolus.

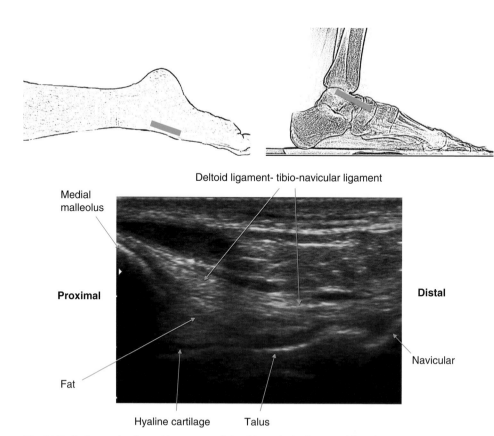

Fig. 4.53. Surface and radiographic anatomy of the tibio-navicular ligament. LS, probe over antero-medial ankle.

Tendons

Tibialis posterior, flexor digitorum longus, flexor hallucis longus from anterior to posterior.

- Tibialis posterior

    Origin – posterior interosseous membrane, tibia and fibula.
    Insertion – navicular.

- Flexor digitorum longus

    Origin – medial posterior tibia.
    Insertion – terminal phalanges lateral four toes.

- Flexor hallucis longus

    Origin – posterior distal fibula.
    Insertion – distal phalanx great toe.

    Posterior tibial nerve: divides into lateral and medial plantar nerves.

- Lateral plantar

    Under flexor retinaculum passes along the sole of the foot to the fifth metatarsal.
    Sensory innervation lateral foot and toes, motor to intrinsic foot muscles.

- Medial plantar

    Under flexor retinaculum to sole. Sensory and motor to medial sole and toes.

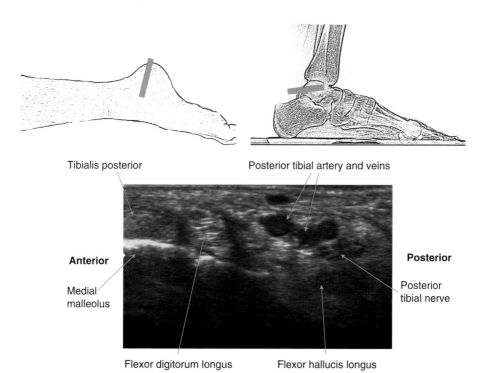

Fig. 4.54. Surface and radiographic anatomy of the tarsal tunnel. TS, probe over medial malleolus. Dynamic examination using foot inversion/eversion.

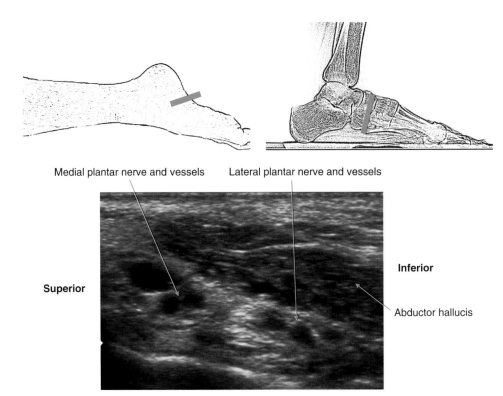

Medial plantar nerve and vessels   Lateral plantar nerve and vessels

Superior

Inferior

Abductor hallucis

Fig. 4.55. Surface and radiographic anatomy of the distal tarsal tunnel. TS, plantar neurovascular bundles in distal tarsal tunnel.

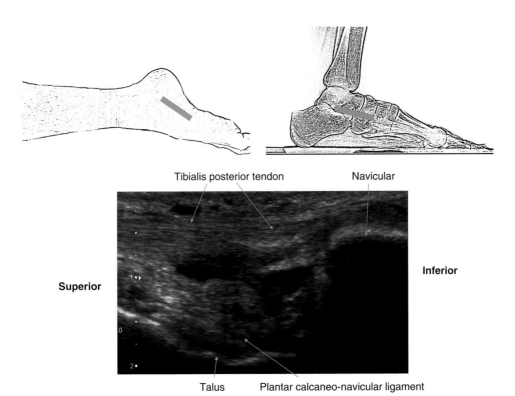

Tibialis posterior tendon   Navicular

Superior

Inferior

Talus   Plantar calcaneo-navicular ligament

Fig. 4.56. Surface and radiographic anatomy of the tibialis tendon. Tibialis posterior tendon. LS, probe over navicular. Distal attachment always appears more ill defined, expanded and hypo-echoic compared to the rest of the tendon.

Ankle: anterior

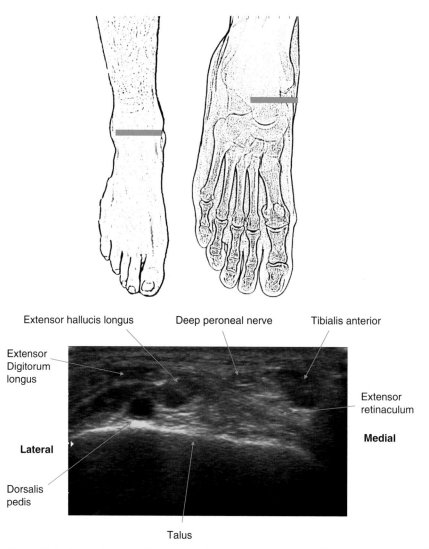

Fig. 4.57. Surface and radiographic anatomy of the extensor retinaculum. TS, probe over anterior ankle.

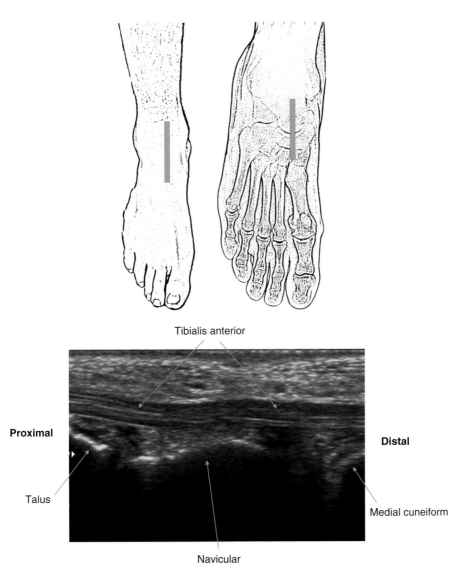

Fig. 4.58. Surface and radiographic anatomy of the tibialis anterior. LS, probe over medial dorsum foot. LS, tibialis anterior tendon insertion. Inserts medial cuneiform and first metatarsal dorsally and medially.

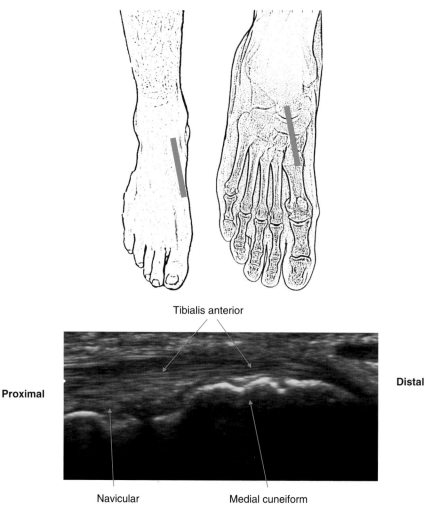

Fig. 4.59. Surface and radiographic anatomy of the tibialis anterior insertion. LS, probe over distal dorsum foot.

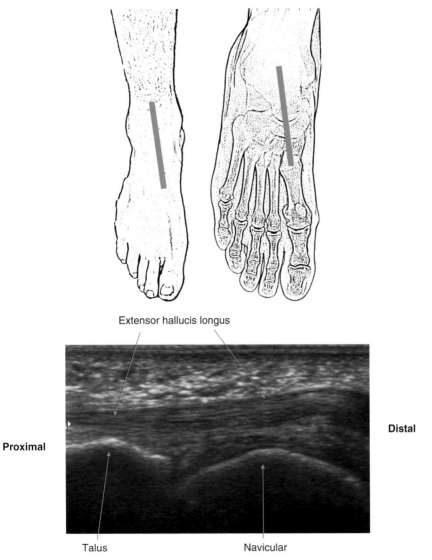

Fig. 4.60. Surface and radiographic anatomy of the extensor hallucis longus tendon. LS, probe over dorsum foot.

Foot

- Plantar surface and sole of foot.

    Web space.

Contents

Flexor digitorum brevis and longus, quadratus plantae, lumbricals, flexor hallucis longus, abductor hallucis, interossei, abductor and flexor digiti minimi.

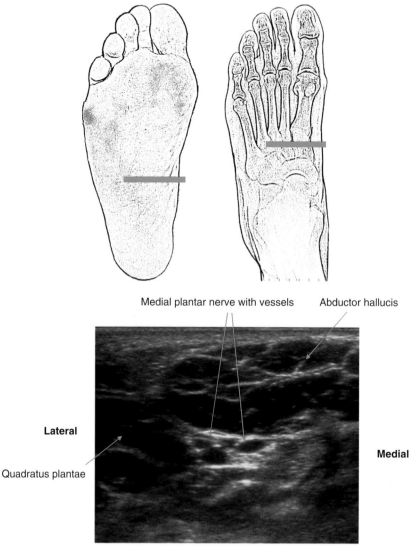

Medial plantar nerve with vessels   Abductor hallucis

Lateral

Medial

Quadratus plantae

Fig. 4.61. Surface and radiographic anatomy of the medial plantar foot. TS, probe plantar aspect foot.

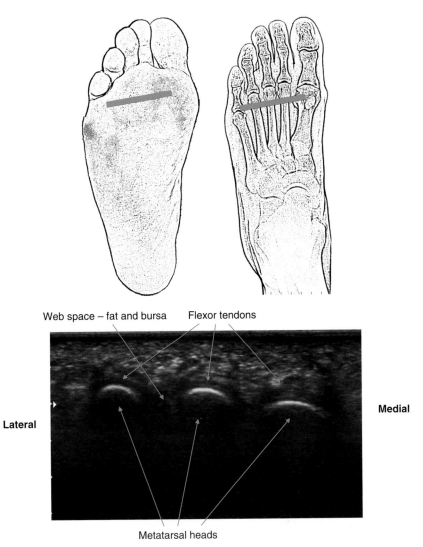

Web space – fat and bursa   Flexor tendons

Lateral

Medial

Metatarsal heads

Fig. 4.62. Surface and radiographic anatomy of the metatarsal heads. TS, probe on plantar surface.

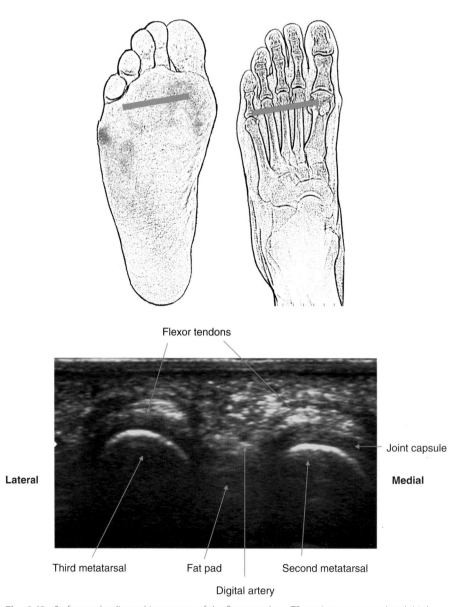

Fig. 4.63. Surface and radiographic anatomy of the flexor tendons. TS, section over second and third metatarsal heads.

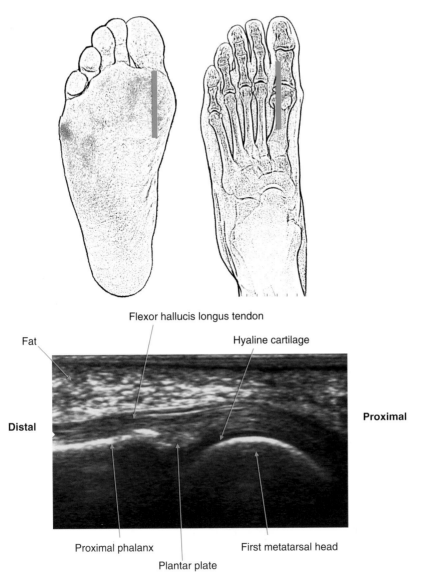

Fat

Flexor hallucis longus tendon

Hyaline cartilage

Proximal

Distal

Proximal phalanx

First metatarsal head

Plantar plate

Fig. 4.64. Surface and radiographic anatomy of the flexor hallucis longus. LS, probe over first metatarsal head. Dynamic examination using flexion/extension of the great toe. LS, flexor aspect toe. Flexor hallucis longus tendon passes distally between the sesamoid bones and inserts in to the distal phalanx of the great toe.

Flexor hallucis brevis

- Origin: medial plantar surface of the cuboid and lateral cuneiform.
- Insertion: splits in two around flexor hallucis longus and inserts either side into the proximal phalanx. Each tendon contains a sesamoid bone.

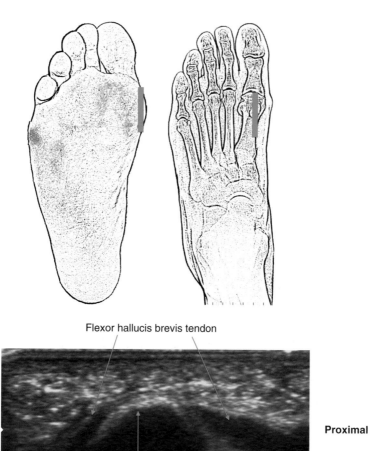

Fig. 4.65. Surface and radiographic anatomy of the medial sesamoid. LS, probe over medial sesamoid.

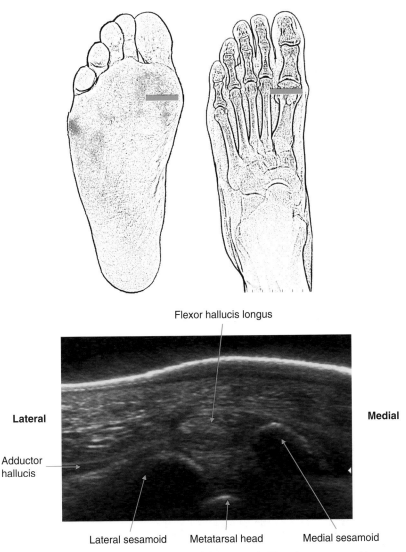

Flexor hallucis longus

Lateral

Medial

Adductor
hallucis

Lateral sesamoid   Metatarsal head   Medial sesamoid

Fig. 4.66. Surface and radiographic anatomy of the sesamoids. TS, probe over sesamoids.

Plantar fascia

Attaches proximally to the medial process of the calcaneum and fans into five slips to merge with the flexor digitorum sheaths to attach to the transverse intermetatarsal ligaments and the base of the proximal phalanges. Strong septa pass from this fascia laterally to divide flexor digitorum from abductor digiti minimi, and medially from abductor hallucis.

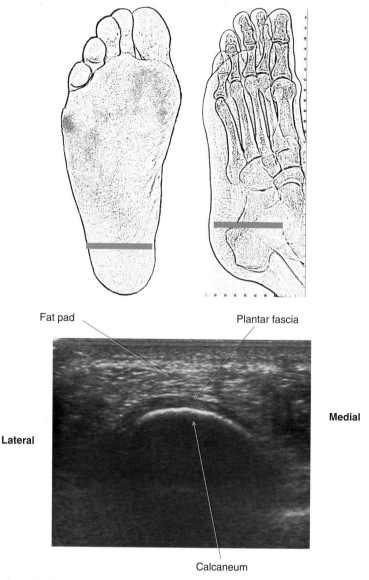

Fig. 4.67. Surface and radiographic anatomy of the plantar fascia. TS, probe over heel pad.

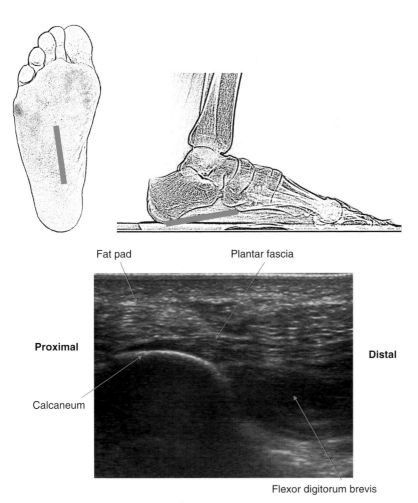

Fat pad   Plantar fascia

Proximal

Distal

Calcaneum

Flexor digitorum brevis

Fig. 4.68. Surface and radiographic anatomy of the plantar fascia. LS, probe midline over plantar surface.

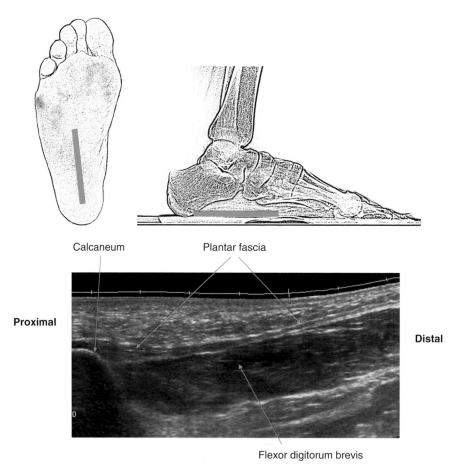

Fig. 4.69. Surface and radiographic anatomy of the plantar fascia. LS, panorama plantar fascia.

Plantar muscles mid foot: four layers

- Superficial: abductor hallucis, abductor digiti minimi, flexor digitorum brevis.
- Second layer: flexor digitorum longus, quadratus plantae, lumbricals, flexor hallucis longus.
- Third layer: flexor hallucis brevis, flexor digiti minimi, adductor hallucis transversus, adductor hallucis obliquus.
- Fourth layer: interossei, tendons of tibialis posterior and peroneus longus.

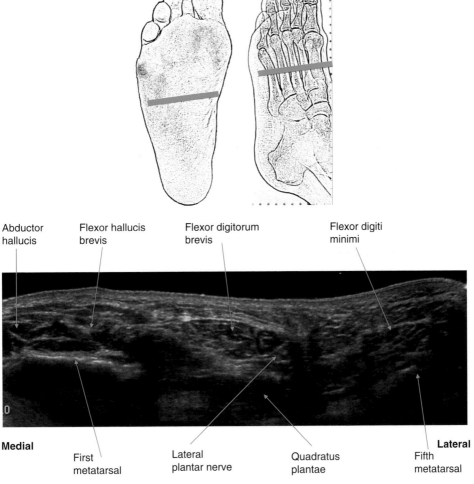

Fig. 4.70. Surface and radiographic anatomy of the plantar muscles. TS, panorama, probe mid foot.

215

Dorsum of foot

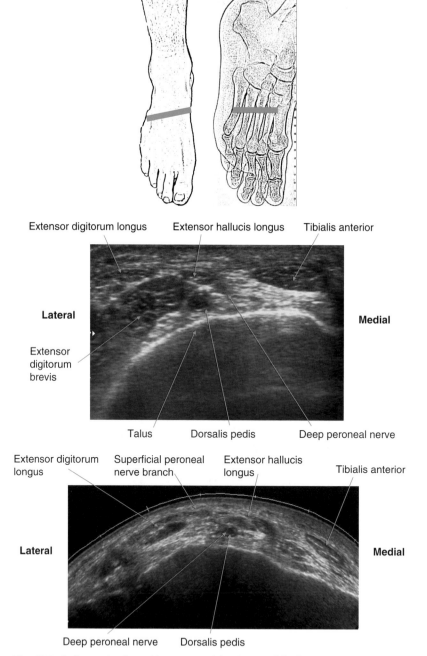

Fig. 4.71. Surface and radiographic anatomy of the dorsum of the foot. TS, probe over mid dorsum of foot. TS, panorama dorsum of foot.

Lisfranc ligament

Ligament from medial cuneiform to second metatarsal base.

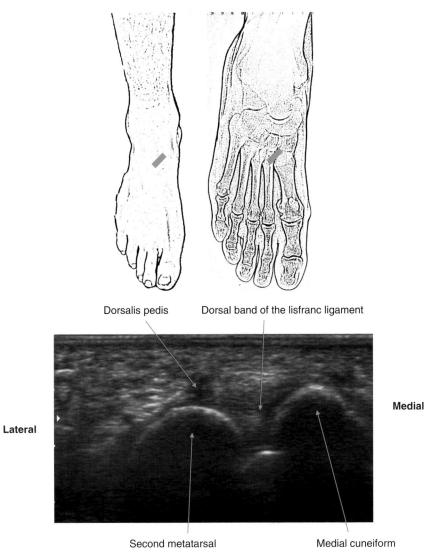

Dorsalis pedis   Dorsal band of the lisfranc ligament

Medial

Lateral

Second metatarsal   Medial cuneiform

Fig. 4.72. Surface and radiographic anatomy of the lisfranc ligament. TS, probe oblique across cuneiform and second metatarsal.

Tibialis anterior

Distal insertion on the navicular and medial cuneiform with some extension along the medial border of the cuneiform.

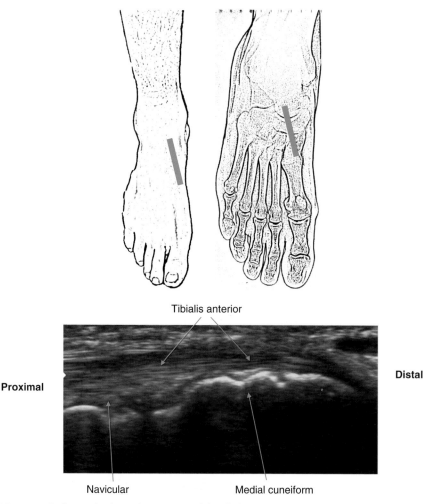

Fig. 4.73. Surface and radiographic anatomy of the tibialis anterior insertion. LS, probe over medial mid foot.

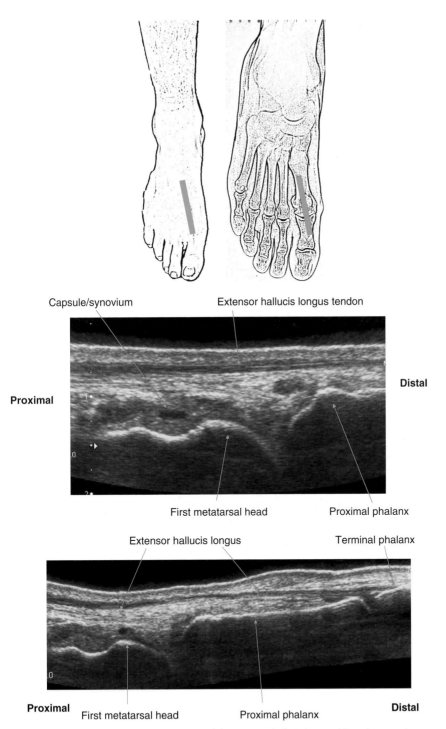

Capsule/synovium

Extensor hallucis longus tendon

Distal

Proximal

First metatarsal head

Proximal phalanx

Extensor hallucis longus

Terminal phalanx

Proximal

First metatarsal head

Proximal phalanx

Distal

Fig. 4.74. Surface and radiographic anatomy of the extensor hallucis longus. LS, probe over dorsum great toe. Dynamic examination using flexion/extension of the great toe. LS, panorama extensor hallucis tendon.

Index

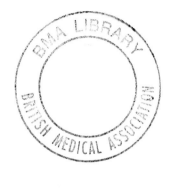